The Jewish East Side
1881-1924

The Library of Conservative Thought

The Jewish East Side
1881-1924

EDITED BY

Milton Hindus

WITH A NEW INTRODUCTION BY THE EDITOR

Transaction Publishers
New Brunswick (U.S.A.) and London (U.K.)

New material this edition copyright © 1996 by Transaction Publishers, New Brunswick, New Jersey 08903. Originally published in 1969 by the Jewish Publication Society of America.

This book is printed on acid-free paper that meets the American National Standard for Permanence of Paper for Printed Library Materials.

Library of Congress Catalog Number: 95-19282
ISBN: 1-56000-842-3
Printed in the United States of America

Library of Congress Cataloging-in-Publication Data

Old East Side.
  The Jewish East Side, 1881-1924 / edited by Milton Hindus ; with a new introduction by the editor.
    p. cm. — (The Library of conservative thought)
  Previously published: The old East Side. Philadelphia : Jewish Publication Society of America, 1969.
  Includes bibliographical references.
  ISBN 1-56000-842-3 (paper : alk. paper)
  1. Jews—New York (N.Y.) 2. New York (N.Y.)—Ethnic relations. 3. Lower East Side (New York, N.Y.)—Ethnic relations. 4. Jews—New York (N.Y.)—Fiction. 5. New York (N.Y.)—Fiction. 6. Lower East Side (New York, N.Y.)—Fiction. 7. American fiction—Jewish authors. I. Hindus, Milton. II. Title. III. Series.
F128.9.J5043 1995
974.7'1004924—dc20   95-19282
                         CIP

dedicated to the memory of

DR. JOSEPH CHESKIS

Dean of Middlesex University and Professor
of Romance Languages and Literature at Brandeis University
which he helped found

and

ESTHER CHESKIS, HIS WIFE

Two marvelous examples of the moral as well as intellectual quality
of the East European Yiddish-speaking immigrants who are celebrated
in some of the following pages

I wish to acknowledge the help I received in preparing this manuscript from my two graduate-student assistants at Brandeis University, Mr. Jack Moskowitz and Mr. Alan Levensohn.

CONTENTS

INTRODUCTION TO THE
TRANSACTION EDITION

Every wave of immigration to the new world came in response to some political event in the old. Persecution brought the Puritans to New England in the seventeenth century. The failed European revolutions of 1848 impelled numbers of German Jews to seek a newer and freer life in the United States. And the assassination of the liberal Russian czar Alexander II in 1881 provoked a reaction in the following years, which caused an exodus from eastern Europe that, in a period of little more than forty years, resulted in a tenfold increase of the Jewish population in the United States, from less than 300,000 in 1870 to over 3,000,000 by the middle of the 1920's. This growth was not without political consequences, the reaction coming from opposite sides of the spectrum, from patriotic organizations that feared for the Anglo-Saxon identity that had established the country's independence and confirmed it in a sanguinary civil war, and from labor unions concerned with disappearing jobs and stagnant or sinking standards of living caused by the competition between sweatshops and native workers who had managed to raise themselves to a somewhat higher economic level. Various and sometimes contradictory pressures brought about the immigration restrictions of 1924, which reversed the traditional policy of welcoming newcomers willing to work at the manifold tasks a growing democracy required for its construction. This period of intersection between the history of the world's Jews and the history of the United States is exceptionally well-documented in journalism, social studies, literature, art, and photography. Its meaning is not only crucial for a better understanding of America and its Jews but, it may now be added, for the origin and growth of the State of Israel as well,

ix

for, without these east European Jews, led by some German Jews of the earlier wave of immigration, such as Louis D. Brandeis, it is unclear if that state would have come into existence, or have long survived if it had done so. This is not to deny or minimize the role of Theodor Herzl, the Austrian Jew who founded the modern Zionist movement, or of Chaim Weizmann, the English Jew who led it successfully to the securing of the Balfour Declaration from Britain. But without the conversion of Brandeis to the new national faith and both the material and moral support of the great majority of American Jews, it is doubtful if Hitler's murderous policy by itself would have sufficed to persuade the United States to recognize and actively support the creation of the first Jewish politically independent commonwealth in the world in almost 2,000 years.

This period of forty years, therefore, clearly has intrinsic as well as collateral claims to close attention and study, and to these claims should be added the fact that the United States, as a result of the vast influx of populations from Asia, Latin America, and elsewhere, appears to be now on the brink, if it is not already in the throes of, another great debate on the subject of immigration, exceeding in intensity anything we have witnessed since the laws of the 1920's temporarily reduced to a trickle the flood that had begun in the last decades of the nineteenth century. Never before, in the seventy years that have passed since then, has the story of those Jewish immigrants, which, for many of us, is the story of our own families and their immediate ancestors, seemed so near or so relevant and possibly instructive with regard to fresh problems with which the country is once more confronted.

It is not that the historical record may be directly helpful to us in anticipating the future, as a philosopher like Santayana encouraged us to believe by suggesting that history might prove less repetitious if only we were capable of learning how to avoid tempting mistakes. Hegel may have been wiser and more pessimistic when he noted sarcastically that the thing we learn from the past is that we do not learn from it. Circumstances are never quite the same, and people (as well as peoples) are always changing; consequently, situations are always new and, in some sense, unprecedented. When immigration restrictions were beginning to be talked about around the time of the First World War, the grateful immigrant Mary Antin, author of *The Prom-*

ised Land, resolutely set her face against those who would shut the gates, invoking her own beautiful experience as well as the promise of the verses of Emma Lazarus inscribed on The Statue of Liberty and welcoming to America the refuse of alien shores. Such eloquent words can never wholly lose their resonance and appeal. They are echoed and supported by the pluralistic philosophy of William James and by his disciple Horace Kallen's moving image of America as an orchestra of many varying cultures and nationalities (in contrast to Zangwill's earlier and more abrasive image of a cruel melting pot). Yet that harmony is increasingly hard for many of us to hear nowadays. It seems more and more like a deafening chaotic cacophony, the pitch of which strains our tolerance to the breaking point. It may not be simply the rigidity of advancing age that suggests that we may be on the verge of some change as momentous as the eighteenth-century revolution that brought our polity into being or the nineteenth-century civil war that tested its ability to survive as an expanding democracy. But the very fact that it can be seriously raised at all is certainly not insignificant.

A native of the Jewish lower east side, born there in 1880, Jacob Epstein must have been among the first to realize its possibilities as an artistic subject and as a sympathetic milieu in which art could be created. When his family became affluent enough to move to a richer section of the city, he retained a studio in the ghetto where he spent most of his time. The first money he earned was from sales to newspapers of sketches he made of interesting types he observed there, and when he was commissioned to do the illustrations for Hutchins Hapgood's book of essays, *The Spirit of the Ghetto,* he realized his dream of going to Europe to study its masterpieces with the masters he found there. Yet, after conquering the world of sculpture, having been knighted by the establishment in England, and fervently admired by leading avant-gardists of the younger generation like Ezra Pound and his friend Hulme, Epstein revisited the scenes of his childhood and youth after a quarter of a century and expressed regret that he had ever left, because the potential of this little corner of America seemed to him the equal of anything he had found elsewhere in the world.

Quite different was the reaction of the expatriate Henry James, who had no such experiences or recollections to guide his sentiments. When he returned to the United States in the early part of the twentieth century after a long absence and was given a tour of what were thought to be interesting developments in the city of New York, which was the scene of some of his early fiction, he saw the newly arrived east Europeans as an invasion of threatening, aggressive, unintelligible Yiddish-speaking barbarians whose coming boded ill for the culture, and even the language of the earlier America he had known. Nothing much of either, he thought, was likely to survive.

In contrast to James's pessimism we have James's great friend, William Dean Howells, whose sympathies were capacious enough to include both James (whom he described as the greatest novelist who ever lived) and a Westerner like Mark Twain, whom he memorably described as "the Lincoln of our literature." After spending some years in Europe (as a consular envoy in Venice during the Civil War), Howells returned, not merely to America but to New York where he discovered its downtown Jews, who he said had a literary taste superior in general to that of the rest of the free-library American public. As a popular novelist, influential critic, and editor, first of *The Atlantic* and then of *Harper's Magazine,* he was strategically in a position to bring to the fore a writer like Abraham Cahan, the editor for fifty years of *The Jewish Daily Forward* and the author of the single best epical description of the East Side in *The Rise Of David Levinsky,* whose earlier novella *Yekl* Howells had touted and compared, not unfavorably, with the work of the brilliant and precocious Stephen Crane.

But the Jewish East Side of New York, in what may be called its heroic period, owes its remembrance not only to artists like Jacob Epstein and writers like Howells, James, and Cahan, but to journalists, photographers, social workers, and reformers and to educators like Morris Raphael Cohen, who taught philosophy to generations of students at The City College (after beginning as an instructor of mathematics in its preparatory school) and to those lecturers in the educational alliances and settlement houses (like Thomas Davidson and Edward King) who guided the first steps of philosophers like Cohen and journalists like Maurice Hindus, who have left memoirs and autobiographies and thematically integrated essays.

A postscript to all this may be found in the self-described "proletarian literature" of Michael Gold, Isidor Schneider, and Samuel

Ornitz. The most impressive and durable artifacts of this period were the least diluted by propaganda and revolutionary agitation but inspired by the ideals of literary craftsmanship, like the works of Charles Reznikoff, Henry Roth, and Anzia Yezierska.

This anthology had its inception in the great multimedia exhibit on the subject of the East Side mounted by The Jewish Museum of New York (housed in a former Warburg residence on Fifth Avenue) in the mid-1960's. This successful show drew an audience of more than 150,000 visitors. The majority of these, according to one observer, consisted of suburbanites who were descendants of the immigrants pictured in the exhibit, moved to self-congratulation on their escape from the miseries of their immediate ancestors.

Much of the material from *The Jewish East Side* was excerpted to serve as part of the catalogue of the exhibit. Some of it clearly originates in the personal history of the compiler. Less obvious may be that it marked a stage in my rediscovery of the work of Charles Reznikoff (1894-1976), who is represented here not by the lyric or narrative modes for which he is known now but by his prose as a novelist and editor in the field of law for which he was professionally trained.

In fact, I have recently returned from San Diego and the annual convention of The Modern Language Association of America where a circle of scholars, critics, poets, and friends celebrated the centenary of his birth with a panel discussion of his work, readings of his poems by poets, and a reception afterwards. Fortuitously, the convention this year was held in close proximity to the Library of the University of California at La Jolla, which had purchased his papers after his death for its Archive for New Poetry. At the meeting of the MLA in San Diego, I learned just how extensive and divergent in many directions the interest in Reznikoff had grown since the time, more than thirty years ago, when it seemed that I had it almost all to myself.

In particular, it reminded me of my lecture in The Jewish Museum, at which Reznikoff himself had been in the audience and in which I discussed his work, the context in which it had been produced, and the enthusiasm with which it had inspired me. It was that very lecture that was credited with the decision of the museum to mount the exhibit, which had long been discussed but not acted upon.

Looking back, after another quarter of a century, with problems of poverty and immigration still looming threateningly on the political horizons of the United States, it may seem that the more things change, the more they remain the same. On the other hand, this gathering of documents, memoirs, and reports, with all their attendant anxieties, trepidations, and anticipations, never realized in fact, may prove heartening and encourage us to think that the present problems of overwhelming magnitude, however insoluble they may seem, are likely, as in the past, to be somehow muddled through without the eruption of such social earthquakes as have afflicted other countries.

In any case, it is useful to be reminded by many of the selections chosen, of the truth in the observation by the Sicilian Prince di Lampedusa (author of one of the most memorable works of twentieth-century fiction, *The Leopard*) that "there are no memoirs, even those written by insignificant people, that do not include social and graphic details of first-rate importance." To which Walt Whitman might have added that in this world where, according to his "Song of Myself," the very weeds have their part to play in what his disciple John Addington Symonds described as "the illimitable symphony of cosmic life," there really are no insignificant people but only those who seem so to the insensitive and the unsympathetic, who are too obsessed with their own concerns and petty ambitions to pay attention to the lives of others.

MILTON HINDUS
April 1995

INTRODUCTION

The monumental outlines of
what may be called the heroic age of lower East Side Jewry in
New York between the 1880's and the mid-1920's could be
drawn in a few broad strokes. Few historians would demur from
tracing the beginnings of the period to a sensational though distant event: the Nihilist assassination of the Russian Czar Alexander II, who had freed the serfs, in Saint Petersburg in 1881,
which triggered a number of anti-Semitic riots among the peasants
and served to rationalize a hostile governmental policy aimed admit-
tedly at driving a third of Russia's millions of Jews out of the
Empire. It ended more than forty years later with the passage of
stringent immigration laws by the American Congress, which
climaxed the efforts after World War I by organized labor and a
variety of professedly patriotic organizations to reverse traditional American policy and to shut the door almost completely
against the unrestricted flow of newcomers into the United States,
particularly those from southern and eastern Europe.

This history, viewed through the narratives of the immigrants
themselves or through those of sympathetic outside observers, is
a sobering spectacle which hardly sustains many romantic myths
later erected upon it. The most honest of those who lived through
it could have said as the cynic did in reply to a question concerning his greatest feat during the French Revolution: "I survived!"
If America appeared to many from far away to be the promised
land, to many others upon nearer view it seemed as if it had to
be reached across a desert. One writer described the New York
he found at the age of fourteen, coming from a small Russian

village, as an "arid zone." This immigrant was exceptional in that he sought as soon as possible to quit the city in order to explore the agricultural world of the American hinterland. Yet even for those who stayed behind in "the wilderness," there was spiritual sustenance corresponding to ancient manna in the form of free education available in public schools, colleges, settlement houses, educational alliance and ethical society, as well as in the lectures of itinerant social philosophers like Thomas Davidson, the precursor of the Fabian Society in England who made the lower East Side of New York the center of his activity in his later years, and Edward King, the old English Chartist who helped broaden the cultural horizons of generations of Jewish immigrants to America.

The Jewish population in this country increased more than tenfold during this period—from a figure of around 300,000 to one of over four millions. In other ways, too, the transformation was startling. Beginning with literally nothing, living in slum tenements in such conditions as to give rise to public scandal, exploited with a cruelty matching the worst that any immigrants to America have ever had to face, substantial numbers of Jews helped themselves to get out from under the burden of poverty in a manner which astonished observers, friendly and less than friendly. The reports of Abraham Cahan as well as of F. Scott Fitzgerald are filled with a sense of romantic wonder at the rapidity of social change in America. The influx transformed radically the internal structure of the American Jewish community. A tiny group in the seventeenth and eighteenth centuries, it had been dominated by Sephardic Jews; later on in the nineteenth century German Jews had become important. Toward the beginning of the twentieth century, Russian and Polish Jews swamped these earlier settlers not only in sheer numbers but eventually in social importance as well.

Not all of the Jews on the lower East Side were immigrants, of course. Jacob Epstein, the sculptor, who was possibly the best known and most distinguished representative of the section in the eyes of the world, was born there in 1880. Ironically enough, this famous native son left the United States early in his twenties to study in Paris and later settled down to work in London, where he was to be singled out for the honor of being knighted. He did not return to the United States for a quarter of a century, and there he felt like a complete foreigner again. His relation to the East Side is perhaps a little like that of James Joyce to Dublin except that it may have been less ambivalent and more affectionate on his side. He felt that he had drawn much of his early material and a lifelong inner strength from this source, and he seems to have regretted somewhat exiling himself from it.

Samuel Johnson suggested to Boswell that Scotland seemed to be a very good place to get away from, and doubtless many East Siders felt the same way at first about their birthplace. The falsification of nostalgia as well as the illumination of it did not come until much later. It is this nostalgia probably which transfigures the literal realism of *The Rise of David Levinsky* and sets it apart completely in aesthetic quality from the works of "the proletarian school" of later decades which were inspired by it. Cahan's story is filled with much more glamour and also with more factual accuracy than the later efforts, which were spoiled for the most part by the propagandistic distortion of life to fit in with the requirements of a political theory.

The most obvious characteristics of life on the lower East Side among the immigrants leaped to the eyes of casual visitor and inmate alike. Social workers, journalists, and youth growing up there were all aware of the same things: abominably crowded homes, people reduced to living in cellars, without windows or light, sleeping in hallways, on roofs or fire-escapes, unbearable heat and stench in summer, unendurable cold in the winter, filth, noise, outdoor plumbing, endless hours of labor for every member of the family down to the smallest, spectacles of vice flaunted for the children to see, bags of refuse flung out of tenement windows onto the hats of citizens passing below, pushcarts, curses, quarrels, vermin of all sorts, rats, beetles as big as half-dollars, street fights and gang warfare.

These images meet us over and over again in all the literature, journalism and tracts on the East Side. Sometimes they appear in the guise of more or less abstract statistics compiled by the social worker, as in Jacob Riis's indictments of the tenement, or in the accounts of compassionate apostles to the poor, like Lillian Wald or Mary Kingsbury Simkhovitch, who started the settlement houses that are an integral part of East Side history, or in the writings of an elementary school teacher like Myra Kelly. Sometimes they come to us in the minutely observant, intelligent and reflective reports of literary men like Howells or journalists like Hutchins Hapgood and Lincoln Steffens. They are present in works of fiction by Cahan, Henry Roth, Charles Reznikoff and Anzia Yezierska. These images are all obviously drawn from the same model.

But despite their importance in building up an impression of what it must have felt like living on the East Side during those hectic decades, one tires of such effects eventually and finds them unrewarding. The description of such environments must always be depressingly the same. Poverty in all times and places, and especially the poverty in metropolitan centers, has been recognized by the same signs and stigmata, whether it is the poverty of ancient Rome described by Juvenal or of contemporary Harlem described by Ralph Ellison. It takes a more penetrating glance to see beneath the surface of the East Side into the disfigurements of its interior life. The chasms between generations there were abysmal. There must always be differences between fathers and children, even in the most unchanging, stable civilizations, but it makes a difference if young people accept 95 per cent of their parents' outlook on the world or if they reject almost the whole of it. The Jewish world of the old East Side resembled that Russian world of the middle of the nineteenth century described by writers like Turgenev in that one part of it lived or tried to live in the Middle Ages, the age of faith, while another segment was slipping toward an anarchic future in which, to quote Fitzgerald's *This Side of Paradise,* "all Gods [were] dead, all wars fought, all faiths in man shaken." The cultural lag was preparing the ground for some terrible social earthquakes in the future.

Some there were fortunate enough to achieve a measure of wisdom despite the handicaps, to overcome their thirst for chaos and destruction, sheer rebelliousness as an end in itself, a sort of permanent revolutionary state of mind. But not all were so lucky, for if tribulations purify the spirit in some cases they overwhelm it in others. Yet the most morbid, introspective accounts of the period cannot wholly hide the fact that for young people, despite everything, the streets were filled with adventure, romance, danger, interest, fascination. There existed an inextricable human mixture of beauty and ugliness in the gang-life, the roof-life, the dock-life, the pigeon-fancying life described by Sholem Asch and others—every kind of life save that of compulsory instruction and the religious cheder, which seemed as hideous and confining to boys as their equivalents had seemed to Mark Twain in the Mississippi Valley long ago.

Not very surprisingly, the deepest views of the scene are the products of the most capacious minds as well as the most sensitive feelings. Schopenhauer once summed up the essence of Kant's transcendental teachings in the statement: "There is no object without a subject." And Proust spelled out the meaning of this thought still more clearly when he said that the world has not been created once and for all but is being re-created anew every time an original pair of eyes looks at it. The difference between literature and journalism could hardly be more graphically illustrated than by comparing Howells' report on the East Side with the writings of Hutchins Hapgood and Lincoln Steffens on the same subject. Hapgood and Steffens were certainly very superior newspapermen both by the standards of their own time and of ours, and the documents which they produced are not without interest and value for all students of the period. Yet the reader cannot help becoming aware of the hopeless limitations of the minds of these authors. Steffens, for example, is consistently lively and amusing, but by jazzing up his most casual observations he somehow manages to create a doubt in the mind of a sensitive reader that things could have taken place in precisely the manner in which he describes them. It is not that he means to mislead us, only that the commonplaceness of his intelligence leads him involuntarily into subtle distortions. To tell the exact truth and to make it credible to the reader without artificial heightening or exaggeration is, as we perceive, an intellectual feat of a higher order than we had imagined.

One of the less kindly reactions to the exhibit devoted to the lower East Side at the Jewish Museum in New York is that it has owed much of its popular appeal to the mood of self-congratulation which it inspires in its visitors. This denigrating hypothesis seems to be susceptible at best only of impressionistic proof, but, assuming that it were correct, is it so objectionable really that, after being exposed to excerpts from museum exhibits of the results of the European holocaust for a generation, Jews in the United States should look back upon their unhappy past with a feeling akin to that of gratefulness? Perhaps, in fact, the emotions it evokes are mixed ones, like those we experience when we see a play like Eugene O'Neill's *Long Day's Journey into Night,* knowing that the end of the play marked only the beginning of the author's own triumphant literary history yet feeling the pathos of what he has shown us about his family life none the less because of this outside knowledge.

As I myself saw it, the show certainly did not encourage a simpleminded nostalgic delight at social progress. There were some strong suggestions there for those capable of responding to them that something may have been lost as well as gained, that material advance has not always been incompatible with spiritual retrogression. It is true, however, that the complexity and ambiguity of the historical process are not recorded as well in the pictorial part of the exhibit as they are in the literary selections of the Catalogue, which the present editor made and which are an abbreviated version of this anthology. There are certain aspects of experience that can only be portrayed in literature, and not even in all kinds of literature equally well. The philosophical and autobiographical essay can obviously come to grips with subjects from the world within man in a way that the drama, by its very nature, finds it difficult if not wholly impossible to do. The graphic arts—painting and photography (which most of the critical observers at the museum agreed was the heart of the exhibit)—are necessarily limited to recording the surfaces of things. They may make interesting patterns or forms out of these surfaces; they may even succeed in suggesting dynamic movement occasionally, ideas, and hidden depths below the surface. But despite the supposedly Chinese proverb that insists that a picture is worth a thousand words, words (as Lessing demonstrated in his classic *Laocoön*) will always be able to do things which no picture, whether taken by the most sensitive camera or cunningly wrought by the hands of a master, can hope to match.

The joys of what it means to be a child growing up anywhere, because the child, like the lyric poet, is able to make a silk purse out of a sow's ear, are captured in the prose of Jacob Epstein's *Autobiography* in a manner which is unique, unforgettable and unequalled even in his own very talented drawings and certainly in photographs. He catches a sense of the old East Side and conveys it to us infectiously as only literature is able to do, because it is in large measure a projection of the artist himself upon the realities around him which the rest of the world saw. Now the latter is the impression recorded upon photographic plate and canvas. It is not to be wondered at that when I spoke in the Catalogue of the "ecstasies" of growing up on the East Side, a critic, who arbitrarily associated my remark with the pictorial side of the show alone, objected that the word was hardly an apt description of what one saw there. I couldn't agree with him more upon this point, but perhaps it is not so bad a description of what the young Jacob Epstein saw, or rather felt, and expressed in eloquent words that, to my mind at least, deserve to belong to American literature and perhaps more particularly to the celebration of a historical period in the city of New York hardly less than do some of the rhapsodic utterances of Whitman on the subject, which evidently served as the inspiration of Epstein.

In the last volume of Proust, the narrator, after reading a pastiche of the *Journal* of the Goncourts which purported to describe in an absolutely fascinating way some of the more stupid and commonplace society people whom he himself had known in life, exclaims in wonder and astonishment: "Magical power of literature! I felt a desire to see the Cottards again, to ask them many details about Elstir, visit the Little Dunquerque shop if still in existence, get permission to go through that mansion of the Verdurins where I had dined." For literature at its best possesses the alchemist's power of transmuting dross into gold. Sometimes it even seems to be capable of making something out of nothing, which is the ultimate reach of creation, and always it is concerned with arresting the fleeting, ephemeral, perishable existences of the phenomenal world and transforming them into something rich and strange, the permanent and indestructible objects of the human imagination. The pen of the artist has precisely this power of making us wish that we, too, had had the privilege of growing up on the East Side and experiencing all the delightful adventures and novelties he describes there. It is with no feeble nostalgia that he summons up an era and a world that have vanished. But in a sense it remains a world that he alone saw and felt and it was hidden from the cameras of Lewis Hine, Jacob Riis and others, no matter how skillful and gifted and resourceful they proved themselves to be.

Nor is the camera or paintbrush capable really of competing with the thoughtful and ironic pages of Howells or with the hunger for wisdom that permeates the words of Morris Raphael Cohen. For these things lie in the province of the written language and nowhere else. Both Howells and Cohen are deceptively simple in appearance and clear-spoken, perhaps because they were so clear-sighted. But their lucidity is complex and subtle, and their words repay rereading, as I myself have found. They do not flaunt their intellectuality and highbrow status in the way that some of our fashionable Jewish contemporaries, who do not have a fraction of the capacity of the older writers, are unfortunately inclined to do.

It may be claimed that the East Side was fortunate in the quality of the interpreters it attracted. Proust remarks somewhere that the drawing rooms of relatively unfashionable hostesses have become famous in literary history, because they were made the subjects of superior memoirs by either the hostesses themselves or some of their talented guests, while some of the most fashionable ones have vanished into oblivion, and it seems to him more or less a matter of chance which of these things has happened. Even some of the journalists reporting the East Side, it has been noted, functioned on a high enough plane to surpass other practitioners of their craft, including some of those who, benefiting from today's added possibilities of publicity, have become better known than their predecessors. This is even more obviously true of a man like Abraham Cahan, who was for fifty years the editor of the largest Yiddish newspaper in the world, the *Jewish Daily Forward*, and was the author of stories and novels which drew the attention and regard of Howells and of other cultivated Americans who were awaiting the advent of a son of the East Side who would imaginatively intercede on behalf of his little section with the larger American world. Cahan was something of an expert juggler both of languages and of literary forms. He wrote almost equally fluently in Russian, Yiddish and English, and his bibliography, which is extensive enough to be printed as a separate book, contains numerous items from all three languages. He shifted easily enough from expository journalism to fictional creation and tactfully respected the characteristics of the different genres he used. If his fiction was not as moving as that of Theodore Dreiser, whose work he admired very much though he opposed Dreiser's Communist ideas resolutely all his life, it was still far above the average level of the American fiction of his period and indeed still seems to me viable for general readers and is something more than a mere document for specialists in immigration problems or in American history.

Some no doubt would see as no matter of blind chance the fact that the mediators on behalf of the East Side should have been so impressive in both quantity and quality, for the section, despite the griminess of its surface (or, perhaps, paradoxically just because of it), attracted observers from the outside with its immense pulsating vitality, its color, its captivating spirit, its seriousness. The same qualities, which were profoundly genuine and not put up for show, also inspired insiders like Cahan. Of a man like Henry Roth, it is perhaps unnecessary to speak here. He is exceptional in a fashion peculiar to the romantic artist. He was possessed by the passion to communicate a vision of the strange life in this country in which he found himself immersed. Basically he may be classified as one of the "proletarian" school, as Professor Walter Rideout has done (his version of the Hebrew melamed is no less of a caricature, despite the cleverness of its drawing, than is Michael Gold's version or Isidor Schneider's or, one is tempted to add, Philip Roth's in such a story as *The Conversion of the Jews*), but the quality that distinguishes him from all the others is the amount of authenticity, the purity of his aesthetic motivation.

T. S. Eliot once said of Henry James that he had a mind so fine it could never be violated by an idea. The seemingly paradoxical statement actually supplies a good clue to the distinction between the real creator and the poster artist. The latter's mind is usually limited so that it is continually being "violated" by his general and abstract ideas. Not all of the proletarians were equally culpable in this respect, to be sure. Schneider is probably the most vulnerable of all, Samuel Ornitz only a little less so. Michael Gold is vigorous and original enough to have inspired some of his comrades for a time, it seems, with suspicions that he was something of a Jewish nationalist, not merely a simulacrum of one. And Edmund Wilson apparently hoped for a time that Gold might develop into an independent creative artist. Joseph Freeman probably comes the closest, in retrospect, to the line which separates tendentiousness from true literature. But none of them makes the transition as successfully as does Henry Roth, who appears to have been a mere hanger-on of the same movement. Roth, one might note, was saved for art by his neuroses, by the very depth of his involvement with himself and his immediate family, which transcended for him all the ideas of Marx and Lenin, the *Daily Worker* and the *New Masses*. The proletarian world-picture is subtly woven into the concluding pages of *Call It Sleep*, but the integrity of the work is not violently twisted out of shape by its message as that of *Jews Without Money* is, unfortunately. Charles Reznikoff's *By the Waters of Manhattan* is even more self-consciously aesthetic than Henry Roth's book, but his day of general recognition has not yet dawned, though there are signs on the horizon of appreciation by a younger generation of American literary men which seem to indicate that this more widespread recognition is bound to come in time.

In a category apart from the journalists, the artists, the literary men, the philosophers, is the sociological observer, exemplified not only by Jacob Riis, Lillian Wald and Mary Kingsbury Simkhovitch, but also perhaps by Howells, for in coming to the East Side, he set aside his character as a popular novelist and the editor of *Harper's Magazine* and assumed the role of the sociologist. The artist, the literary man, and the journalist are all intrigued by the variety in the spectacle of life and with the problems of communicating their sense of it to others. They do not, insofar as they are true to themselves and their vocations, set themselves up as moralists or judges of the phenomena they report. The world to them is a world they never made and do not really feel responsible for. It moves them by its mere existence, by its rhythms and shifting forms, but the response elicited is instinctual rather than intellectual.

The student of society, on the other hand, though there is occasionally an ideal of scientific objectivity which inspires his investigations and makes for an attitude of cool detachment from the situation of the human beings whom he describes, is usually moved by other considerations. The mainspring of the settlement house workers' psychology is probably compassion and humanitarianism. They went to live among the poor for the same reason that their counterparts in the populist movements in Czarist Russia around the same period went out to "the dark people." The social worker had a vision of what the desirable average level of existence in a good society ought to be, felt himself or herself to have reached that level or even, because of unearned privileges of birth and education, to have surpassed that level, and desired to raise the poor and underprivileged up to it. The immigrant Jew fifty, sixty, and seventy years ago in this country appealed to the generous impulses of such people much as the Negroes do today. It is true that condescension and heavy-handedness in the approach of some of these people—like that unnamed tactless librarian at the Educational Alliance, described in Maurice Hindus' memoir of the period, *Green Worlds*—offended the self-esteem of those whom they wished to help, but the ones who have left a mark in history and are in this book, we may safely assume, did not belong to this category. About some of these figures there was a quality of almost religious fervor, self-abnegation, sympathy, and inexhaustible kindness, which in another age might have made them candidates for canonization.

Jacob Riis is not so much a dispassionate student of society as a would-be improver of it, a reformer, who differs from the more radical or revolutionary specimens of his type only in his greater effectiveness, which is due to his acceptance of the assumptions of the democratic republic in which he found himself and the courage, patience and fortitude with which he worked through established institutions to bring about change. He did not make the error of so many others of trying to destroy existing social forms "root and branch" and to substitute new, untried, or impractical devices for them.

Riis was a hard-boiled newspaper editor and political figure. He had known hardship and misery himself as an immigrant from Denmark equal to those encountered by any of the people he wrote about. He was not disposed, therefore, to be sentimental about their lot as were some of those who, because of their own origins and softer life in the upper classes of conventional society, were almost traumatically shocked by what they found on the East Side. His camera pitilessly recorded some of the most interesting and valuable studies we have of immigrant life. One memorable picture which he snapped of a bearded Jewish workingman in a coal-cellar preparing for the Sabbath has been particularly singled out for praise and comment by more than one admiring observer. When it came to writing about the East Side, Riis was so natural and unaffected that he did not trouble to hide or disguise his own ethnic bias against his subjects, which transpires through every line of his famous book *How the Other Half Lives*. A satiric witticism has it that the Jews are just like other people, only more so. Something like that seems to have been the feeling of Riis. If America in general appeared to him money-mad, the poverty-stricken Jews were even more deluded than the rest of the population. The children, of course, were a different matter, and his treatment of them is altogether more sympathetic than his description of their elders. But Riis was moved to action not by what he felt for the poor primarily (though he was insulted in his dignity as a human being by the contemplation of the conditions under which they had to exist) but by what he felt was due to his own good citizenship as an American. It was for America's sake that he wanted to raise the standards of living of the poor. It is the strange, eccentric mixture of his individualistic attitudes, I think, that made him effective as a pleader. He was so obviously sincere in what he said, even to the point of frankly expressing his antipathies, that no one could regard him as being anything but inner-directed; he was nobody's man but his own. He was no propagandist or lobbyist, no retained attorney or group spokesman. He said what he thought at all times fearlessly, without favor to anybody, and so his words carried an added weight.

Howells was cut from another bolt of cloth. He, too, had known what it was to be poor, though never as poor as the Danish immigrant Riis. He was not born a Boston Brahmin but was only an adopted son. His unusual talents had opened the doors of opportunity to him early, but he was a social dreamer with a much more Utopian bent to his character than the practical-minded Riis. He was also the possessor of a finer, more subtle intelligence and disposed of a much greater literary power and eloquence. The Jews of New York, particularly the poor Jews of the lower East Side, interested him because he saw in them a leaven for the inert mass of unintellectual Americans who surrounded him most of his life (he had served the United States in a diplomatic post in Europe for a time), and these Americans of coarser fiber irritated him only to a slightly lesser degree than they irritated his friends Henry James and Mark Twain.

The Jews interested him in part because they carried the intellectual aura of Europe with them, for Howells was a lover of Europe and things European, including in particular its realistic literature, a taste for which he almost despaired at times of making popular in romantic America, though it was naturally popular among the Jews who had been brought up on the great novel literature of the nineteenth century in Russia. It is this which inspired the bitter reflection he recorded in *Harper's Magazine* in 1915, which Van Wyck Brooks quotes in his biography of Howells: "With us the popular taste is so bad, so ignorant, so vulgar, that it suggests the painful doubt whether literacy is a true test of intelligence and a rightful ground of citizenship. . . . We will go a little further and say that the literary taste of the Russian Jews on the East Side is superior to that of the average native American free-library public." The Jews were also for him the People of the Book, and he could not altogether shake off, as he looked at them, the idea of their relationship to Christ and his disciples. Despite the realism of his critical stance, he was much more visionary than a man like Riis. One of the consequences of Howells' intellectuality was his search for the weaknesses and falsifications of familiar popular stereotypes—the very thing which had contented the simpler Riis and to which the latter had added his own mite of first-hand observation. For example, I suppose that no adjective has stuck more persistently to the word Jew than the word "dirty," and so Howells emphasizes the extraordinary degree of hygienic cleanliness which he had found in his personal observations of the ghetto. Howells is an intellectual and therefore almost by definition not inclined to accept any formulations of the truth save his own.

Not so Riis. He is an independent man but he is also a simple one, who believes in the basic soundness of proverbial wisdom. He is satisfied when he can confirm, on the basis of his own experience, the validity of what other people have thought of a subject. I must say this seems to me far from a contemptible motivation and more likely, by and large, to be productive of common sense than many a self-anointed intellectual's insistence upon originality of approach, even in situations the least likely to afford this quality scope. Such an insistence often results in mere perversity, eccentricity and insignificance. Yet Riis's can be a somewhat menacing virtue; its very directness may result in crudity and insensitivity; its lack of the critical spirit implies a certain absence of self-consciousness, too. It may beget self-contradiction, which is either unnoticed or flaunted with bravado as an unsuspected merit. Riis did not escape these dangers. His contribution, on both social and literary grounds, is more shadowed and flawed by ambiguities than he himself realized, but perhaps for this very reason, the raw documentation of his observations and attitudes remains one of the most important historical quarries for the period in question.

One Gentile observer of the East Side, whose antipathy for the people there was expressed in a much more elegant style than that of Jacob Riis, is the novelist F. Scott Fitzgerald. In his novel *The Beautiful and Damned,* published in 1922, a trip by the hero, Anthony Patch, down Manhattan by the elevated trains of the period is described as follows: "Down in a tall busy street he read a dozen Jewish names on a line of stores; in the door of each stood a dark little man watching the passers from intent eyes— eyes gleaming with suspicion, with pride, with clarity, with cupidity, with comprehension. New York—he could not dissociate it now from the slow, upward creep of this people—the little stores, growing, expanding, consolidating, moving, watched over with hawk's eyes and a bee's attention to detail—they slathered out on all sides. It was impressive—in perspective it was tremendous."

The tone of this passage toward its subject (concentrated in such a verb as "slathered") is unfortunately as representative of the work of Fitzgerald himself as it is of the time in which he wrote. One critic has suggested that Fitzgerald merely displaced his own Irish self-hatred with contempt for one of the other minorities in America. This is an interesting hypothesis, but it is a demonstrable fact that anti-Jewish attitudes were widespread and rather fashionable in the 1920's in America (the decade in which Ford's *Dearborn Independent* published *The Protocols of the Elders of Zion* and the *Saturday Evening Post* editorially commended Stoddard's racist "classic," *The Rising Tide of Color*). In the nineteenth century philo-Semitism predominated in America, as we can see in reading Longfellow, Whitman, Bryant, Whittier, Howells and Mark Twain, but toward the end of the century and increasingly in the first third of the twentieth century a very different and more hostile attitude came to the fore. Early examples of it are to be found in Henry Adams, Henry James and Edith Wharton, later examples in Ezra Pound, T. S. Eliot, Fitzgerald, Dreiser, Mencken, Thomas Wolfe, and E. E. Cummings. The cause of this "backlash" is not hard to find. Increasing Jewish numbers, affluence and influence produced an effect similar to the one which they produced long ago upon the Pharaoh "who knew not Joseph." Aeschylus in *Agamemnon* has Clytemnestra say: "Who feareth envy feareth to be great!" From the remotest times to the most recent (as one can see in the unabashed confessions of an anti-Semitic French writer of genius, Louis-Ferdinand Céline) envy has probably been the principal source of feeling against the Jews, and this feeling, existing amorphously in society at large, eventually finds expression in literature.

Oddly enough, the effect of Hitler's unparalleled atrocities has been (thus far at least in American literature) to obliterate almost entirely the anti-Semitism which was so chic in the earlier part of the century that traces of it can be found even in a writer like Gertrude Stein, whose rootless cosmopolitanism did not prevent Wyndham Lewis from referring to her as "a brilliant Jewish lady." Hitler's holocaust seems to have separated those who were pathological on the subject of the Jews (like Pound and Céline) from those, like Eliot and Fitzgerald, who were more conventional and less possessed. Fitzgerald in the late 1930's seemed to be horrified (as Thomas Wolfe was, too) by the consequences which anti-Semitic ideas were leading to in Germany. Such people either retracted some of their earlier statements about the Jews or fell silent altogether on the subject. Now, at the beginning of the last third of the twentieth century, however, it ought to be recalled perhaps that there was a time earlier in the century when writers like Robert Frost and some others appeared to be quite exceptional among their American contemporaries in that their work did not contain at least some pages offensive to the sensibilities of their Jewish fellow citizens.

In this anthology, I have limited myself to material which was initially in the English language and excluded translations. This decision has cut me off from the voluminous work about the East Side in Yiddish and the less extensive literature in Hebrew. No one is more aware than I am of what this has entailed. Some years ago, in the magazine *Jewish Heritage* in an article which dealt with the relationship between Howells and Cahan, I had occasion to note the importance of Cahan's Yiddish memoirs and to deplore the fact that they were not available in the English language. Until that time, only a few pages from these monumental and fascinating five volumes had appeared in English in the pages of a learned journal. The entire laborious project has recently been tackled, though it is far from being completed. Yet even if its results were available to me for selection, I very much doubt if, faced with a choice between the translated *Pages out of My Life* and the novels *Yekl* or *The Rise of David Levinsky*, which were both originally conceived and executed in the English language by Cahan himself (with a stylistic felicity which inspired the praise of Howells), I should choose the former. I have made no exceptions in the application of this rule even in the case of a poet like Morris Rosenfeld, some of whose lyrics have appeared in English in several different versions since Professor Leo Weiner of Harvard discovered them for the English-speaking world in 1898. The lyric impulse does not cross linguistic barriers readily even in the case of the most celebrated poets like Goethe and Heine. It is hardly a reflection, therefore, on Rosenfeld himself or on his well-intentioned translators to say that his thoughts (in some of his prose as well as in his verses) sound a little anachronistic in the garb of a language alien to him. In general, I should add, I have striven as much as possible to eliminate as many selections as I could in which a documentary interest was not combined with a literary one. Obviously, this has not always proved to be feasible. It has indeed been one of my principal objects in this book to supply evidence of the fact that the East Side has not only left an imprint upon American life, upon Jewish life and Jewish literature in this country, but also upon American literature and culture.

As yet, there is no single authoritative book to pull the diverse history of the East Side together. Perhaps there never will be. Yet there is a certain wealth of materials, both documentary and literary, that deal with the subject, and it is some specimens of these materials that are offered in this anthology. Even the most humble writers of autobiography or of autobiographical fiction describing the immigrant period make one think of a touching democratic thought voiced by the Sicilian Prince di Lampedusa, who was himself the author of an unretouched autobiography and of a remarkable biographical fiction entitled *The Leopard*: "There are no memoirs, even those written by insignificant people, which do not include social and graphic details of first-rate importance." Walt Whitman would have probably gone even further and added that in this world and scheme of creation where, according to *Song of Myself*, even the weeds have their proper place and part to play in what John Addington Symonds called "the illimitable symphony of cosmic life," there really are no insignificant people but only those who seem to be so to the unkind, the unsympathetic, or those too busy or preoccupied with their own concerns to pay attention to others.

Elsewhere, I have spoken of the East Side as "a great proving ground for Americans," an experience which "separated the wheat from the chaff, the men from the boys." In saying this, I had in mind the observation made by Joseph Conrad and by Hemingway that every experience in life which hurts and wounds without wholly destroying us in the end only succeeds in making us stronger. The East Side, except for a few artists like Epstein and a lot of children who were growing up there, was generally speaking for the older generation an ordeal, a transition, a painful initiation, a trauma which accompanied passage from the old-world shtetl to the sense of a privileged new nationality and status which has come to American Jews in the last fifty years or so. Other Americans have been produced out of other crucibles. The East Side was an individual but not unique historical phenomenon, and this writer sees no reason for apologizing for the sense of relief which one feels that the period of adjustment to a new civilization lies behind the Jews of America rather than before them. None of us, as Tolstoy indicated in *War and Peace,* is wise enough to predict the future, either individual or collective, with any real confidence in our correctness, but the results of the past that are already in, even granting all the imperfections of materialism, ostentation and vulgarity in suburbia which a host of critical spirits has highlighted, are not such as to inspire us with any legitimate feeling of fear or pessimism.

JACOB EPSTEIN

In 1945, when Jacob Epstein was sixty-five years old, he was described by *Current Biography* as "probably the best-known contemporary sculptor as well as the most discussed artist since Rodin."

He was born on Hester Street, the heart of the lower East Side of New York, the third child in a large family of Russian-Polish Jews. As his *Autobiography* indicates, he enjoyed growing up in the New York of the 1880's. When his family became affluent enough to move uptown, he retained a room on the East Side which he used as a studio. In addition to public schooling, he was able to pick up a pretty good literary education on his own.

His talent for art showed itself early, and he pursued studies at the Art Students League in New York City. In 1901, he went to work in a foundry for bronze sculpture and at the same time studied sculptural modelling under a distinguished sculptor, George Grey Barnard. A turning point in his life came when he met the well-known journalist Hutchins Hapgood, who commissioned him to do a series of drawings for his collection of articles about the ghetto entitled *Spirit of the Ghetto*. It is undoubtedly due in part to these drawings that Hapgood's book has been reprinted more than once in recent years. Epstein received the sum of $400 for his contribution to Hapgood's book. That was a sizable sum in those days and, together with his earnings from some drawings which he sold to the *Century Magazine*, it enabled him to realize his ambition to go to Europe for further studies at several art academies.

Though his ultimate goal in going to Europe was Paris, there

1

appears to have been a brief sojourn first in England where, according to Arthur Strawn, he lived in an old stable on rice and tea. He had come, however, at a propitious moment when "rebels were just beginning to gain recognition at the expense of the Academicians." In Paris, he studied at the *École des Beaux Arts* and at the Julian Academy. He won some important prizes, but the life in England and the character of the people attracted him back there to make his home. In 1906, he married a "charming and forceful" Scotswoman, Margaret Gilmour Dunlop. The couple was very impecunious at the beginning, occupying two bare rooms of which one served as a studio. To earn money, Epstein served as a model at an art school, posing three nights a week from six o'clock until ten and earning $1.50 a night!

In 1907, Epstein won his first important public recognition in England when Queen Alexandra, consort to King Edward VII, purchased his bronze *Head of an Infant*. That spring, too, on the recommendation of the etcher Muirhead Bone, he was commissioned by the architect Charles Holden to decorate the new British Medical Association Building. Like almost all of his work, this one became the subject of a public controversy, which gave him a notoriety that was certainly preferable to obscurity but which troubled him a good deal. Later on, he wrote: "I do not see myself as a martyr, but what has always astonished me was the bitterness of the attacks on my statues."

He naturally fell in with the avant-garde of the period in England, which included some influential expatriates from America like Ezra Pound and T. S. Eliot. Pound wrote an early, sensitive, discerning appreciation of Epstein's work. This was an experimental period in Epstein's life which brought him into relationship with the Vorticist movement. Epstein's unfinished sculpture *Rock-Drill* impressed Pound so much that it may account for the title of a group of his *Cantos* many years afterward. The outstanding intellectual figure in this pre-World War I group was T. E. Hulme, and he appreciated Epstein's work most of all. As a matter of fact, he wrote the first book about Epstein, the manuscript of which was unfortunately lost when he was killed in battle in 1917.

The first published work about Epstein was Bernard van

Dieren's *Epstein* (1920). Many signs of esteem and recognition of his work came from outstanding and influential figures in the art world over the years. H. R. Wilenski wrote of him: "Even the purist must bow down before Romantic art of this compelling intensity." But Epstein himself is evidently at variance with the category to which he has here been assigned, for he has written: "I have always sought the deeply intimate and human and so wrought them that they became classic and enduring."

Among his large works were the tomb he sculpted for Oscar Wilde in Père Lachaise Cemetery in Paris and the Memorial to W. H. Hudson in Hyde Park in England. He created striking portraits in stone and bronze of some of the best known men in the world in his time: Joseph Conrad, Winston Churchill, George Bernard Shaw, Albert Einstein, John Dewey, and many political figures, like Ramsay MacDonald and Ernest Bevin, whose fame has dwindled with time. These capture unforgettable images of their subjects. Conrad, who addressed Epstein as "Master," said to a friend that, in sitting for him during the last months of his life, he felt that he was being transmitted to posterity in the likeness which was destined to be remembered best. The same could be said of many others of his works. The technique he used in these portraits has been compared to that of Rodin in his famous bust of Balzac. Epstein's work, however, appears to this observer to be more realistic in the best sense of the word, less mannered, violent and distorted for purposes of symbolism, than this example of the French master's work.

Precisely how much Epstein suffered from the controversies that swirled around his work most of his life is indicated by the bitter, almost Juvenalian invective of the following passage: "How superficial is the world of art, and what a wretched lot of logrollers, schemers, sharks, opportunists, profiteers, snobs, parasites, sycophants, camp followers, social climbers and 'four-flushers' infest the world of art—this jungle into which the artist is forced periodically to bring his work and live." He was once described as "a big and powerful man radiating enormous vigor and the impression of almost inexhaustible physical energy. His torso is huge, his neck strong; his grey eyes are sad, his sensitive tortured lips never quite still. He suggests at once Michelangelo and William Blake." Socially, he made an excellent impression, too. He was a well-informed conversationalist who did not monopolize the conversation. He loved music to distraction, especially the work of Bach and Beethoven. While he was engaged in his own work, he said that he did not care who was Prime Minister or what the weather was like. His freedom from vanity is perhaps indicated by the fact that he never answered his fan mail. He died "old and full of honors" in 1959, one more illustration of the observation that those who begin by rebelliously blasting the foundations of art may end under the dome of immortality. Whether officially sanctioned or not (and Epstein, despite the knighthood conferred on him by the British, steadfastly denied that his work had ever received the suffrage of the Establishment in art), his immortality seems as certain, at this moment, as that of any man of his century. And perhaps his writings, which are too few in number, will participate in the attention which is generally given to him, his work, and his personality.

Autobiography

My earliest recollections are of the teeming East Side where I was born.

This Hester Street and its surrounding streets were the most densely populated of any city on earth, and looking back at it, I realise what I owe to its unique and crowded humanity. Its swarms of Russians, Poles, Italians, Greeks, and Chinese lived as much in the streets as in the crowded tenements, and the sights, sounds, and smells had the vividness and sharp impact of an Oriental city.

Hester Street was from one end to the other an open-air market, and the streets were lined with push-carts and pedlars, and the crowd that packed the side-walk and roadway compelled one to move slowly.

As a child I had a serious illness that lasted for two years or more. I have vague recollections of this illness and of my being carried about a great deal. I was known as the "sick one." Whether this illness gave me a twist away from ordinary paths, I don't know, but it is possible. Sometimes my parents wondered at my being different from the other children, and would twit me about my lack of interest in a great many matters that perhaps I should have been interested in, but just wasn't. I have never found out that there was in my family an artist or anyone interested in the arts or sciences, and I have never been sufficiently interested in my "family tree" to bother. My father and mother had come to America on one of those great waves of immigration that followed persecution and pogroms in Czarist Russia and

Selection from Jacob Epstein's *Autobiography*, published by the Hulton Press, London, 1965. Also by E. P. Dutton in the United States.

Poland. They had prospered, and I can recall that we had Polish Christian servants who still retained peasant habits, speaking no English, wearing kerchiefs and going about on bare feet. These servants remained with us until my brother Louis, my older brother, began to grow up; and then with the sudden dismissal of the Polish girls, I began to have an inkling of sexual complications. My elder sister, Ida, was a handsome, full-bosomed girl, a brunette, and I can recall a constant coming and going of relatives and their numerous children. This family life I did not share. My reading and drawing drew me away from the ordinary interests, and I lived a great deal in the world of imagination, feeding upon any book that fell into my hands. When I had got hold of a really thick book like Hugo's *Les Misérables* I was happy, and would go off into a corner to devour it.

I cannot recall a period when I did not draw, and at school the studies that were distasteful to me, Mathematics and Grammar, were retarded by the indulgence of teachers who were proud of my drawing faculties, and passed over my neglect of uncongenial subjects. Literature and History interested me immensely and whatever was graphic attracted my attention. Later, I went to the Art Students' League up town and drew from models and painted a little, but my main studies remained in this quarter where I was born and brought up. When my parents moved to a more respectable and duller part of the city, it held no interest for me whatever and I hired a room in Hester Street in a wooden, ramshackle building that seemed to date back at least a hundred years and, from my window overlooking the market, made drawings daily. I could look down upon the moving mass below and watch them making purchases, bartering, and gossiping. Opposite stood carpenters, washerwomen, and day-workers, gathered with their tools in readiness to be hired. Every type could be found here, and for the purpose of drawing, I would follow a character until his appearance was sufficiently impressed on my mind for me to make a drawing. A character who interested me particularly was a tall, lean, and bearded young man, with the ascetic face of a religious fanatic, who wandered through the streets lost in a profound melancholy. His hair grew to his shoulders, and upon this was perched an old bowler hat. He

6

carried a box in one hand, and as he passed the push-carts, the vendors would put food into his box, here an apple, there a herring. He was a holy man and I followed him into synagogues, where he brooded and spent his nights and days.

On one occasion I was taken to see the Chief Rabbi, a man of great piety, who had been brought from Poland to act as the Chief Rabbi; but as New York Jews do not acknowledge a central authority, he never attained this position. An attempt to use him to monopolize the kosher meat industry was indignantly rejected. This sage and holy man lived exactly as he would in a Polish city, with young disciples, in ringlets (*payis*), who attended him as he was very infirm, lifting him into his chair, and out of it, and solicitous of his every movement. The patriarchal simplicity of this house much impressed me. The New York Ghetto was a city at that time transplanted from Poland. Parallel with all this was the world of the "intelligentsia," the students, journalists, scholars, advanced people, socialists, anarchists, freethinkers, and even "free lovers." Newspapers in Yiddish, Yiddish theatres, literary societies, clubs of all kinds for educational purposes, night-classes abounded, and I helped to organize an exhibition of paintings and drawings by young men of the quarter. There existed a sort of industry in enlarging and colouring photographs, working them up in crayon, and there were shops that did a thriving trade in this. I had student friends who, to earn money, put their hands to this hateful work, and by industry could earn enough to go on with more serious studies. I never had to do this, as I could always sell my drawings.

I kept the room on Hester Street until on returning to it one morning I found it burnt to the ground, and my charred drawings (hundreds of them) floating about in water with dead cats. I had to find another room, this time in a tenement with clothing workers, where I restarted my studies. I never remember giving up this second room, and perhaps because of that it has returned to me in dreams with a strange persistence; even in Paris and in London, in my dreams I find myself in the room as I left it, filled with drawings of the people of the East Side.

The many races in this quarter were prolific, children by hundreds played upon the hot pavements and in the alleys. Upon the

7

fire-escapes and the roofs the tenement dwellers slept for coolness in summer. I knew well the roof life in New York, where all East Side boys flew kites; I knew the dock life on the East and West Sides, and I swam in the East River and the Hudson. To reach the river the boys from the Jewish quarter would have to pass through the Irish quarter, and that meant danger and fights with the gangs of that quarter: the children of Irish immigrants.

The Jewish quarter was on one side bounded by the Bowery, and this street at that time was one long line of saloons, crowded at night by visitors to the city, sailors, and prostitutes. As a boy I could watch through the doors at night the strange garish performers, singers and dancers; and the whole turbulent night-life was, to my growing and eager mind, of never-ending interest. I recall Steve Brodie's saloon with its windows filled with photographs of famous boxers, and the floor inlaid with silver dollars. A tour along the Bowery, for a boy, was full of excitement, and when you reached Chinatown, crooked Mott Street, leading to Pell Street, you could buy a stick of sugarcane for one cent and, chewing it, look into the Chinese shop windows, and even go into the temple, all scarlet and gilding, with gilded images. The Chinamen had a curious way of slipping into their houses, suddenly, as into holes, and I used to wonder at the young men with smooth faces like girls. Chinese children were delightful when you saw them, although no Chinese women were to be seen. Along the West Front, on the Hudson side, you saw wagons being loaded with large bunches of bananas, and great piles of melons. Bananas would drop off the overloaded wagons; you picked them up, and continued until you came to the open-air swimming baths with delightful sea water. I was a great frequenter of these swimming places, and went there until they shut down in November for the winter.

New York was at this period the city of ships of which Whitman wrote. I haunted the docks and watched the ships from all over the world being loaded and unloaded. Sailors were aloft in the rigging, and along the docks horses and mules drew heavy drays; oyster boats were bringing their loads of oysters and clams, and the shrieks and yells of sirens and the loud cries of overseers made a terrific din. At the Battery, newly arrived immigrants, their shoulders laden with packs, hurried forward, and it must have been with much misgiving that they found their first steps in the New World greeted with the hoots and jeers of hooligans. I can still see them hurrying to gain the Jewish quarter, and finding refuge amongst friends and relatives. I often travelled the great stretch of Brooklyn Bridge, which I crossed hundreds of times on foot, and watched the wonderful bay with its steamers and ferry-boats. The New York of the pre-skyscraper period was my formation ground. I knew all its streets and the water-side, I made excursions into the suburbs; Harlem, Yonkers, Long Island, and Coney Island I knew well, and Rockaway where I bathed in the surf. I explored Staten Island, then unbuilt on, and the palisades with their wild rocks leading down to the Hudson river.

Early on I saw the plastic quality in coloured people, and had friends amongst them, and later was to work from coloured models and friends, including Paul Robeson, whose splendid head I worked from in New York. I tried to draw Chinamen in their quarter, but the Chinese did not like being drawn and would immediately disappear when they spotted me. The Italian Mulberry Street was like Naples, concentrated in one swarming district. Within easy reach of each other, one could see the most diverse life from many lands, and I absorbed material which was invaluable.

At this time I was a tremendous reader, and there were periods when I would go off to Central Park, find a secluded place far away from crowds and noise, and there give myself up to solitary reading for the day, coming back home burnt by the sun and filled with ideas from Dostoyevsky's *Brothers Karamazov,* or Tolstoy's novels. Also I absorbed the New Testament and Whitman's *Leaves of Grass,* all read out of doors, amongst the rocks and lakes of the Park. It was only later I read the English poets, Coleridge, Blake, and Shelley, and still later Shakespeare. During my student days at the League, I would drop into Durand Ruel's gallery on Fifth Avenue, and there see the works of many of the Impressionist painters, which were not so sought after in those days. I saw splendid Manets, Renoirs, and Pissarros, and Durand Ruel himself, noticing my interest, gave me special opportunities to see pictures which went back to Europe and are now in the Louvre and National Gallery. I was very well acquainted at this time with the work not only of the American artists who were influenced by the Impressionists, but also with the works of the older men who now constitute the "Old Masters" of America— Winslow Homer, George Innes, Homer Martin, Albert Ryder, and Thomas Eakins. The sincerity of these men impressed me, and my boyhood enthusiasms have been justified by time.

I began to feel at this period that I could more profoundly express myself, and give greater reality to my drawings by studying sculpture. I had been drawing and reading to excess, sometimes in dim light, and my eyes had suffered from the strain, so that sculpture gave me relief, and the actual handling of clay was a pleasure.

Naturally my family did not approve of all that I did, although they saw that I had what might be called a special bent. My turning to sculpture was to them mysterious. Later they could not understand why I did certain things, any more than do the critics who profess to see in me a dual nature, one the man of talent, and the other the wayward eccentric, the artist who desires to *épater*. What chiefly concerned my family was why I did things which could not possibly bring me in any money, and they deplored this mad or foolish streak in me.

They put it down to the perversity that made me a lonely boy, going off on my own to the woods with a book, and not turning up to meals, and later making friends with Negroes and anarchists.

My grandmother on my father's side was a cantankerous old creature who swore that we children were going to the dogs, and were *goyim*, and she continued travelling between Poland and New York, as she declared she would not die in a pagan land; but—alas! for her wish—it was in New York she died.

My grandparents on my mother's side were a dear old couple, whose kindness and patriarchal simplicity I remember well. Every Friday evening the children would go to them to get their blessing. Before the Sabbath candles they would take our heads in their hands and pronounce a blessing on each one of us in turn. Then followed gifts of fruit and sweets. I was one of a large family, a third child, and my elder brother Louis was at all times sympathetic and helpful. Of my brothers, Hyam was an exceptionally powerful youth, a giant of strength, headstrong and with a personality that got him into scrapes. My sister, Chana, a beautiful, fair-haired girl, with a candid, sweet nature, was a great favourite of mine, and we often went out together. My father and mother in the evenings would lie in bed reading novels in Yiddish; my father would read aloud, and I often stayed awake listening to these extravagant romances. Saturday in the synagogue was a place of ennui for me, and the wailing prayers would get on my nerves, and my one desire would be to make excuses to get away. The picturesque shawls with the strange faces underneath only held my attention for a short while; then the tedium of the interminable services would drown every other emotion. Certainly I had no devotional feelings, and later, with my reading and free-thinking ideas, I dropped all practice of ceremonial forms, and as my parents were only conventionally interested in religion, they did not insist. I was confirmed at the age of thirteen in the usual manner, but how I ever got through this trying ordeal I cannot now imagine. The Passover Holidays always interested me for the picturesque meal ceremonies, and I remember my father, who was "somebody" in the synagogue, bringing home with him one of the poor men, who waited outside to be chosen to share the Passover meal. These patriarchal manners I remember well, although there was about them an air of bourgeois benevolence which was somewhat comic. The earnestness and simplicity of the old Polish Jewish manner of living has much beauty in it, and an artist could make it the theme of very fine works. This life is fast disappearing on contact with American habits, and it is a pity that there is no Rembrandt of to-day to draw his inspiration from it before it is too late.

My parents did not discourage me, but could not understand how I could make a living by art. Their idea of an artist was that of a person who was condemned to starvation. Sculpture became to me an absorbing interest. When I started seriously to work I felt the inadequacies of the opportunity to study. For one thing, only a night class existed in New York, and also there was very little antique sculpture to be seen; modern sculpture hardly existed. I longed to go to Paris, and my opportunity came when I

11

met Hutchins Hapgood, the writer, who was very interested in the East Side, and asked me to illustrate a book which he had written about it. I drew for him the poets, scholars, actors, and playwrights, and also made some drawings of the people.

I remember well the great actor Jacob Adler, at whose flat I called to make a drawing of him. He was surrounded by a houseful of dependents of all kinds, apart from his numerous family, and the confusion and excitement were immense. Finding a clean collar out of bags that contained hundreds of collars took up most of the time. Adler had a head like those you see in Japanese prints, long and white, and heavy, chameleon-like eyelids. This Jewish actor had a court, and when you saw him in the streets he was preceded and followed by his fans. He lived in public. I also drew Jacob Gordin, who wrote plays about Jewish life which had a strong Ibsenish flavour. He was a heavy, bearded man, whom I recall reading to an audience one of his plays, sitting informally at a table, smoking a cigar.

In their dressing-rooms, I drew Kessler the actor, also Moscowitch, and the poets Lessin and Moritz Rosenfeld, who had spent his early life in tailors' shops.

I was known in the market, and wherever I took up a position to draw I was looked upon sympathetically, and had no difficulty in finding models. Jewish people look upon the work of an artist as something miraculous, and love watching him, even though they may be extremely critical. I sometimes think I should have remained in New York, the material was so abundant. Wherever one looked there was something interesting, a novel composition, wonderful effects of lighting at night, and picturesque and handsome people. Rembrandt would have delighted in the East Side, and I am surprised that nothing has come out of it, for there is material in New York far beyond anything that American painters hunt for abroad.

I took this East Side drawing work very seriously, and my drawings were not just sketches. With Gussow, my Russian artist friend, I drew the life of the East Side, and one or two other artists joined us, so that we might have developed a School had we kept on. Since then I know of no one except John Sloan and George Luks who were inspired by New York life.

I should like to recover some of these drawings I made of East

Side life, but I understand they were dispersed in sales, and perhaps destroyed. I also drew for periodicals, and the Century Company purchased drawings from me. I could have remained in America and become one of the band, already too numerous, of illustrators, but that was not my ambition, and at the school I felt something of a fish out of water. The art students' life was distasteful to me. I could not join in their rags and their beer, and their bad jokes got on my nerves. Nevertheless, there were students who purchased my studies from the model for a dollar or two, and I was especially friendly with James Carrol Beckwith, an American painter who was the drawing teacher at the League. He was sympathetic to me, and very interested in what I told him and showed him of the East Side life, which to the up-towner was like the life of the jungle for strangeness.

A great friend was James Kirk Paulding, a man of fine literary discernment, and a friend of Abraham Cahan, the editor of *The Forward*. Paulding was in the habit of reading to four or five of us boys on a Sunday morning, and this was my first introduction to Conrad's work. In this way I heard *The Nigger of the Narcissus* and *Typhoon*, also most of Turgeniev. I attended concerts of symphonic music, and went to the Metropolitan Opera House and heard Wagner's *Ring*, naturally from the gallery, miles away from the stage. Also I went to political meetings where I heard Prince Kropotkin and Eugene Debs, also Henry George, the Single Taxer. I observed, drew a great deal, and dreamed a great deal more. In connection with political meetings and what would now be called "left wing" sympathies and friends, I was an observer only, and never a participator, as my loyalties were all for the practice of art, and I have always grudged the time that is given to anything but that. This is not to say that I am a believer in the "ivory tower" theory. On the contrary, a wide knowledge of men and events seems to me necessary to the artist, but participation and action in political events and movements must remain a matter of personal predilection. In this connection I think of Courbet, whose life was embittered and whose work suffered because of the part he took in the Commune.

My people were not, as has been stated, poor. On the contrary, they were fairly well off, and as the family was large I saw a great deal of Jewish orthodox life, traditional and narrow. As my thoughts were elsewhere, this did not greatly influence me, but I imagine that the feeling I have for expressing a human point of view, giving human rather than abstract implications to my work, comes from these early formation years. I saw so much that called for expression that I can draw upon it now if I wish to.

As we are living in a world that is changing rapidly, I may be compelled to modify this attitude and plump for direct participation and action.

I was not altogether a city boy, and excursions to the country outside New York bred in me a delight in outdoors. In this connection I well remember that one winter my friend Gussow and I hired a small cabin on the shores of Greenwood Lake, in the State of New Jersey. In this mountain country I spent a winter doing little but tramping through snow-clad forests, cutting firewood, cooking meals and reading. To earn a little money we both helped to cut the ice on the lake, this work lasting about two weeks. This was very hard but congenial work, as we were taken to the ice-fields by sledges drawn by a team of horses in the early morning over the hard-frozen lake, and returned in the evening on the sledges, when we saw wonderful snow views of mountain sides ablaze with sunset colours. It was a physical life full of exhilaration and interest. At this place lived a couple with whom I became very friendly, a Mr. and Mrs. Wells. This Mr. Wells made photographs of visitors for a living during the summer, and in the winter he painted. His wife, a little Welsh woman, had psychic powers, and she prophesied a great future for me, so Wells informed me. This couple were looked upon by the villagers as queer. They were the only persons in the place who took an interest in art or in anything but village life. It was rather a degenerate place altogether, where there had been a great deal of inbreeding, as only three family names existed.

After this winter at Greenwood Lake I determined to work at sculpture. I entered a foundry for bronze casting and attended a modelling class at night at the League. George Grey Barnard was the teacher. The class was mostly made up of sculptors' assistants, and we had to have some ardour to put in an evening's modelling after a hard day's work in ateliers and workshops. Barnard would come one evening of the week to give us criticisms, but he rarely got through a full class of students. He

14

would look at the study and give you a penetrating glance (he had a cast in his eye), and then start his talk, in which he would usually lose himself for the rest of the evening. The students would gather round him, and as he was a man of great earnestness, he was very impressive. Barnard was ascetic in his habits, and hated the notion that his students drank or were at all Bohemian: later when I was to meet him in London and lunch with him, he thought it was a concession, as he was on holiday, to let me have wine. I knew his early work, and at that time he was the only American sculptor one could have any respect for.

I met Tom Eakins, but as a sculptor he impressed me as being too dry and scientific, and I looked forward to the day when I would be able to see the ancients and Rodin. I longed to see originals of Michelangelo and Donatello, and Europe meant the Louvre and Florence.

There has been a tremendous impetus given to American sculpture since I was a boy in New York, and numerous commissions are given to sculptors, but of the lasting value of this renaissance of sculpture I am unable to judge from here. Mountains have been carved, and on reading of these tremendous-sounding events, I imagined that I might have played a part in all this, but it was another destiny that called me, and I have had to create heroic works from time to time in my studio, without commissions and with little or no encouragement from official bodies.

Native American sculptors did not give one much inspiration, and at that time no one thought of Mexican or pre-Columbian Indian work. The fact was, the interest in early American Continental sculpture came from Europe. By a sort of reaction American artists now try hard to be American.

My desire now was to get to Paris. With the money from my drawings for Hapgood's book I bought a passage for France. I can recall, with the unthinking heedlessness of youth, climbing the gangway to the vessel that was to take me away from America for a period of twenty-five years. When I reached the top of the gangway, my mother ran after me and embraced me for the last time.

One night, in March, 1913, in Paris, I dreamed of my mother, and immediately received news of her early death.

15

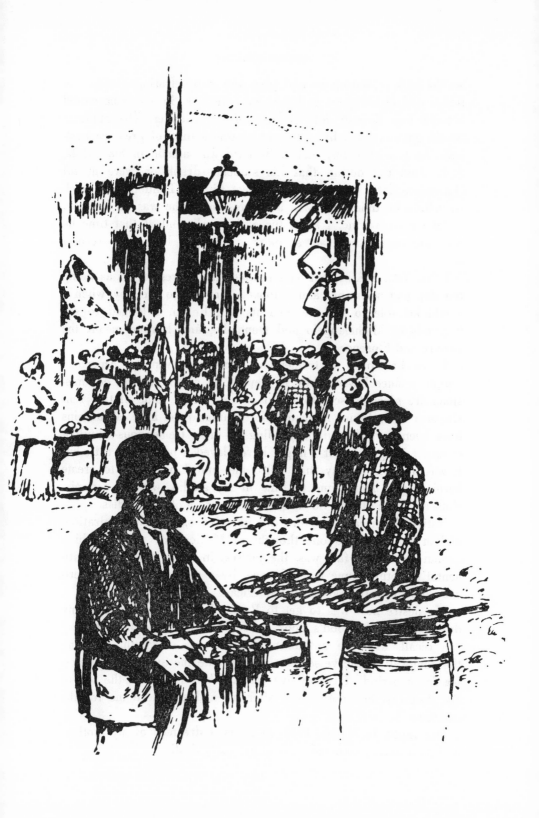

ABRAHAM CAHAN

Abraham Cahan was born in Russia on July 7, 1860. He came to America in 1882. In its obituary of him in 1951, the *New York Times* described him as a Socialist leader, novelist, critic and newspaperman who, for many years, had been an outstanding figure of New York's East Side.

"For nearly six decades, as teacher, organizer and journalist, he occupied a major position among the poor and laboring masses of his own people, contributing profoundly to their Americanization and adjustment in the American scheme of things. . . . A Russian revolutionist at twenty, a successful American novelist at thirty, editor of a moribund little Socialist Yiddish daily at forty, he became the dominant force of the greatest Jewish daily in the world at fifty, a position which he occupied to the end of his life. Wherever Yiddish is spoken, Mr. Cahan's name was known as the editor of *The Jewish Daily Forward.* . . . In his literary sketches and novels he wrote with art and understanding of the life and toil of these masses. . . . In his everyday work as a newspaperman and labor spokesman he contributed materially to the elimination of the sweatshop and the elevation of the living and cultural standards of his own people and the working people as a whole. . . . He was born near Vilna of poor Orthodox parents. His father wanted him to be a rabbi. . . . In 1880, he graduated from the Teachers Institute of his native city and for a while taught in a governmental school. Early in his youth he became interested in the revolutionary movement, and at the age of twenty-one was compelled to flee Russia. In 1882, he arrived in New York penniless. For a while he worked in a cigar factory. He was one of the founders of the first Socialist society and founded the first Jewish union in this country. In 1885 he founded the *Neue Zeit* and shortly afterwards was instrumental in starting the New York *Arbeiter Zeitung* in association with Morris Hillquit."

His literary career, as distinguished from his journalistic one, began at the *Forward,* according to his autobiography, but his interest in literature had begun to develop much earlier. It was his wife who drew his attention to the psychological profundity of Tolstoy's *Anna Karenina.* He read that book and reread it; Chekhov's *Crimean People* also affected him very much. It was under the influence of these Russian authors that he began to appraise his own experiences in terms of their suitability and potential as writing material. Among English-language authors he notes having read early in his career George Eliot, Dickens, Thackeray, Hawthorne, Howells, Henry James, Byron, Shelley, and Wordsworth.

He notes his preference for Howells to James because of what he felt was the former's greater resemblance to the Russian literature which he admired. He was, however, also aware very early, it seems, of Howells' weaknesses: a too great mildness of temperament and Puritanical modesty and decorum. In 1892, before Cahan had attempted the work that was to give him importance in English as well as in Yiddish, Howells was curious enough to meet him and was impressed by the fact that the editor of a socialist newspaper in a language which even its own readers and speakers did not respect was widely read in English and American literature as well as in Russian.

Cahan began by translating some of his own Yiddish stories into English. The first was called *A Providential Match* (which was later to give a title to a book of his stories). After being rejected by *Harper's Monthly,* it was accepted by a magazine called *Short Stories,* where apparently it was read accidentally by Howells' wife, who brought it to her husband's attention. This was in February 1895. In June of the same year, Cahan's *Sweat-Shop Romance* appeared in the same magazine. Howells invited him to his home, and Cahan was encouraged to show him a novella, which he had written and called *Yankel, the Yankee.* The older novelist read it, liked it, and suggested shortening the title to *Yekl.* Again, Cahan's story was rejected at *Harper's.* The ground stated by the fiction editor was that its readers were "not interested in the Jewish East Side." Cahan notes that in the late 1880's, the expression "American Jewish literature" was beginning to make itself heard but was treated as a joke.

Howells was persistent, however, for he believed in both Cahan and his book and he suggested that Cahan take it to a friend, Ripley Hitchcock, literary advisor to the publishing firm of Appleton and Company, who were the publishers of Stephen Crane, whom Howells had also "discovered." Appleton accepted the book and published it in July 1896. In general, *Yekl* was favorably received by the press. The *New York Times* praised its realism and local color. The *Sun* compared it favorably with Charles Dudley Warner's writing on the same section and with Stephen Crane's New York story *George's Mother.* It concluded that Cahan's portraits were better than those found in the other books, because his were less stereotyped and more interesting. Howells had privately praised the naturalness of the book, its authenticity, and Cahan's handling of the language. But Cahan was astonished when Howells went further and composed a feature critical article for the *New York World* in which he hailed Cahan and Stephen Crane as twin stars of a rising new school of realists in American fiction. This article was very favorably received by the public and was reprinted widely all over the United States. Overnight, Cahan was famous in the English-speaking world, which no Yiddish writer before him had ever succeeded in penetrating. A newspaper syndicate did a feature article about him and he was invited to fashionable literary gatherings in the most select company. On September 22, 1896, he was one of the guests of honor at the Lanthorn Literary Club in New York, sharing the platform with Hamlin Garland and Stephen Crane. In May 1897, the novel was published by Heinemann in England. *Cosmopolitan Magazine* signed a contract with him and published his short story "Circumstances."

Despite these remarkable successes, however, Cahan sadly notes that *Yekl* did not really sell well: "The 'immoral' love-story of two poor Jewish immigrants did not interest the reading public."

Cahan's *succès d'estime* did have important consequences nevertheless in the sense that it opened up the English-language press in America to him. Difficulties at the *Forward* led him for a time to abandon Yiddish journalism completely and to go to work for Lincoln Steffens and the *Commercial Advertiser*. There he met Hutchins Hapgood and was the invisible "guide, philosopher and friend" who helped him thread his way through the mysteries of the ghetto, which no outsider had fathomed before him. Cahan himself wrote reports on East Side life for a large number of American newspapers and magazines before returning to the *Forward* on his own terms. Moses Rischin, who is preparing a full-scale biography of Cahan, believes that the experience at the *Commercial Advertiser* was the crucial watershed of Cahan's career. From that time on, he was never very far from the mainstream of American life and letters. It is not necessary to speak here of his later accomplishments. These are reasonably well known to close students of American literature, though a writer like Ludwig Lewisohn felt that Cahan's talent in such a work as *The Rise of David Levinsky* had never yet received its proper due as art among the critics and historians of this literature. Periodically, other men, like the late Isaac Rosenfeld, have added their audible voices to this judgment, so that one feels that, sooner or later, it is bound to prevail among the knowledgeable and cultivated.

It may be added that under Cahan's direction the *Forward* became such a political power in New York that it was able to break Tammany's hold on the lower East Side and send the first socialist, Meyer London, to Congress. In 1933, however, Cahan was expelled from the Socialist party because he supported Roosevelt for President.

It is not the least of Cahan's contributions to culture that in the pages of the *Forward* he published such Yiddish writers as I. J. Singer, Zalman Schneour, and Sholem Asch before the general reading public had ever heard of them. Cahan is one of those rare figures of whom it may truly be said that though he owed much to the people and section which singled him out as its literary representative, that people and section also owed a great deal to him. No one could have filled his part quite as adequately as he did. Had he never lived or had he never come to America, in my estimation, it would have made quite a difference to the East Side and in a measure to the United States.

Yekl

It was after seven in the evening when Jake finished his last jacket. Some of the operators had laid down their work before, while others cast an envious glance on him as he was dressing to leave, and fell to their machines with reluctantly redoubled energy. Fanny was a week worker and her time had been up at seven; but on this occasion her toilet had taken an uncommonly long time, and she was not ready until Jake got up from his chair. Then she left the room rather suddenly and with a demonstrative "Good-night all!"

When Jake reached the street he found her on the sidewalk, making a pretense of brushing one of her sleeves with the cuff of the other.

"So kvick?" she asked, raising her head in feigned surprise.

"You cull dot kvick?" he returned grimly. "Good-bye!"

"Say, ain't you goin' to dance to-night, really?" she queried shamefacedly.

"I tol' you I wouldn't."

"What does *she* want of me?" he complained to himself proceeding on his way. He grew conscious of his low spirits, and, tracing them with some effort to their source, he became gloomier still. "No more fun for me!" he decided. "I shall get them over here and begin a new life."

After supper, which he had taken, as usual, at his lodgings, he went out for a walk. He was firmly determined to keep himself from visiting Joe Peltner's dancing academy, and accordingly he took a direction opposite to Suffolk Street, where that establish-

A chapter from *Yekl* by Abraham Cahan, published by Appleton and Company, New York, 1896.

ment was situated. Having passed a few blocks, however, his feet, contrary to his will, turned into a side street and thence into one leading to Suffolk. "I shall only drop in to tell Joe that I cannot sell any of his ball tickets, and return them," he attempted to deceive his own conscience. Hailing this pretext with delight he quickened his pace as much as the overcrowded sidewalks would allow.

He had to pick and nudge his way through dense swarms of bedraggled half-naked humanity; past garbage barrels rearing their overflowing contents in sickening piles, and lining the streets in malicious suggestion of rows of trees; underneath tiers and tiers of fire escapes, barricaded and festooned with mattresses, pillows, and featherbeds not yet gathered in for the night. The pent-in sultry atmosphere was laden with nausea and pierced with a discordant and, as it were, plaintive buzz. Supper had been despatched in a hurry, and the teeming populations of the cyclopic tenement houses were out in full force "for fresh air," as even these people will say in mental quotation marks.

Suffolk Street is in the very thick of the battle for breath. For it lies in the heart of that part of the East Side which has within the last two or three decades become the Ghetto of the American metropolis, and, indeed, the metropolis of the Ghettos of the world. It is one of the most densely populated spots on the face of the earth—a seething human sea fed by streams, streamlets, and rills of immigration flowing from all the Yiddish-speaking centres of Europe. Hardly a block but shelters Jews from every nook and corner of Russia, Poland, Galicia, Hungary, Roumania; Lithuanian Jews, Volhynian Jews, south Russian Jews, Bessarabian Jews; Jews crowded out of the "pale of Jewish settlement"; Russified Jews expelled from Moscow, St. Petersburg, Kieff, or Saratoff; Jewish runaways from justice; Jewish refugees from crying political and economical injustice; people torn from a hard-gained foothold in life and from deep-rooted attachments by the caprice of intolerance or the wiles of demagoguery-innocent scapegoats of a guilty Government for its outraged populace to misspend its blind fury upon; students shut out of the Russian universities, and come to these shores in quest of learning; artisans, merchants, teachers, rabbis, artists, beggars—all come in

23

search of fortune. Nor is there a tenement house but harbours in its bosom specimens of all the whimsical metamorphoses wrought upon the children of Israel of the great modern exodus by the vicissitudes of life in this their Promised Land of to-day. You find there Jews born to plenty, whom the new conditions have delivered up to the clutches of penury; Jews reared in the straits of need, who have here risen to prosperity; good people morally degraded in the struggle for success amid an unwonted environment; moral outcasts lifted from the mire, purified, and imbued with self-respect; educated men and women with their intellectual polish tarnished in the inclement weather of adversity; ignorant sons of toil grown enlightened—in fine, people with all sorts of antecedents, tastes, habits, inclinations, and speaking all sorts of subdialects of the same jargon, thrown pell-mell into one social caldron—a human hodgepodge with its component parts changed but not yet fused into one homogeneous whole.

And so the "stoops," sidewalks, and pavements of Suffolk Street were thronged with panting, chattering, or frisking multitudes. In one spot the scene received a kind of weird picturesqueness from children dancing on the pavement to the strident music hurled out into the tumultuous din from a row of the open and brightly illuminated windows of what appeared to be a new tenement house. Some of the young women on the sidewalk opposite raised a longing eye to these windows, for floating by through the dazzling light within were young women like themselves with masculine arms round their waists.

As the spectacle caught Jake's eye his heart gave a leap. He violently pushed his way through the waltzing swarm, and dived into the half-dark corridor of the house whence the music issued. Presently he found himself on the threshold and in the overpowering air of a spacious oblong chamber, alive with a damp-haired, dishevelled, reeking crowd—an uproarious human vortex, whirling to the squeaky notes of a violin and the thumping of a piano. The room was, judging by its untidy, once-whitewashed walls and the uncouth wooden pillars supporting its bare ceiling, more accustomed to the whir of sewing machines than to the noises which filled it at the present moment. It took up the whole of the first

24

floor of a five-story house built for large sweat-shops, and until
recently it had served its original purpose as faithfully as the four
upper floors, which were still the daily scenes of feverish industry. At the further end of the room there was now a marble soda
fountain in charge of an unkempt boy. A stocky young man with
a black entanglement of coarse curly hair was bustling about
among the dancers. Now and then he would pause with his eyes
bent upon some two pairs of feet, and fall to clapping time and
drawling out in a preoccupied sing-song: "Von, two, tree! Leeft
you' feet! Don' so kvick—sloy, sloy! Von, two, tree, von, two,
tree!" This was Professor Peltner himself, whose curly hair, by the
way, had more to do with the success of his institution than his
stumpy legs, which, according to the unanimous dictum of his male
pupils, moved about "like a *regely* pair of bears."

The throng showed but a very scant sprinkling of plump
cheeks and shapely figures in a multitude of haggard faces and
flaccid forms. Nearly all were in their work-a-day clothes, very
few of the men sporting a wilted white shirt front. And while the
general effect of the kaleidoscope was one of boisterous hilarity,
many of the individual couples somehow had the air of being
engaged in hard toil rather than as if they were dancing for
amusement. The faces of some of these bore a wondering martyr-
like expression, as who should say, "What have we done to be
knocked about in this manner?" For the rest, there were all sorts
of attitudes and miens in the whirling crowd. One young fellow,
for example, seemed to be threatening vengeance to the ceiling,
while his partner was all but exultantly exclaiming: "Lord of the
universe! What a world this be!" Another maiden looked as if she
kept murmuring, "You don't say!" whereas her cavalier mutely
ejaculated, "Glad to try my best, your noble birth!"—after the
fashion of a Russian soldier.

The prevailing stature of the assemblage was rather below
medium. This does not include the dozen or two of undergrown
lasses of fourteen or thirteen who had come surreptitiously, and—
to allay the suspicion of their mothers—in their white aprons. They
accordingly had only these articles to check at the hat box, and
hence the nickname of "apron-check ladies," by which this truant
contingent was known at Joe's academy. So that as Jake now

25

stood in the doorway with an orphaned collar button glistening out of the band of his collarless shirt front and an affected expression of *ennui* overshadowing his face, his strapping figure towered over the circling throng before him. He was immediately noticed and became the target for hellos, smiles, winks, and all manner of pleasantry: "Vot you stand like dot? You vont to loin dantz?" or "You a detectiff?" or "You vont a job?" or, again, "Is it hot anawff for you?" To all of which Jake returned an invariable "Yep!" each time resuming his bored mien.

As he thus gazed at the dancers, a feeling of envy came over him. "Look at them!" he said to himself begrudgingly. "How merry they are! Such *schnoozes,* they can hardly set a foot well, and yet they are free, while I am a married man. But wait till you get married, too," he prospectively avenged himself on Joe's pupils; "we shall see how you will then dance and jump!"

Presently a wave of Joe's hand brought the music and the trampling to a pause. The girls at once took their seats on the "ladies' bench," while the bulk of the men retired to the side reserved for "gents only." Several apparent post-graduates nonchalantly overstepped the boundary line, and, nothing daunted by the professor's repeated "Zents to de right an' ladess to the left!" unrestrainedly kept their girls chuckling. At all events, Joe soon desisted, his attention being diverted by the soda department of his business. "Sawda!" he sang out. "Ull kin's! Sam, you ought ashamed you' selv; vy don'tz you treat you' lada?"

In the meantime Jake was the centre of a growing bevy of both sexes. He refused to unbend and to enter into their facetious mood, and his morose air became the topic of their persiflage.

By-and-by Joe came scuttling up to his side. "Goot-evenig, Dzake!" he greeted him; "I didn't seen you at ull! Say, Dzake, I'll take care dis site an' you take care dot site—ull right?"

"Alla right!" Jake responded gruffly. "Gentsh, getch you partnesh, hawrry up!" he commanded in another instant.

The sentence was echoed by the dancing master, who then blew on his whistle a prolonged shrill warble, and once again the floor was set straining under some two hundred pounding, gliding, or scraping feet.

"Don' be 'fraid. Gu right aheat an' getch you partner!" Jake went on yelling right and left. "Don' be 'shamed, Mish Cohen. Dansh mit dot gentlemarn!" he said, as he unceremoniously encircled Miss Cohen's waist with "dot gentlemarn's" arm. "Cholly! vot's de madder mitch *you?* You do hop like a Cossack, as true as I am a Jew," he added, indulging in a momentary lapse into Yiddish. English was the official language of the academy, where it was broken and mispronounced in as many different ways as there were Yiddish dialects represented in that institution. "Dot'sh de vay, look!" With which Jake seized from Charley a lanky fourteen-year-old Miss Jacobs, and proceeded to set an example of correct waltzing, much to the unconcealed delight of the girl, who let her head rest on his breast with an air of reverential gratitude and bliss, and to the embarrassment of her cavalier, who looked at the evolutions of Jake's feet without seeing.

Presently Jake was beckoned away to a corner by Joe, whereupon Miss Jacobs, looking daggers at the little professor, sulked off to a distant seat.

"Dzake, do me a faver; hask Mamie to gib dot feller a couple a dantzes," Joe said imploringly, pointing to an ungainly young man who was timidly viewing the pandemonium-like spectacle from the further end of the "gent's bench." "I hasked'er myself, but se don' vonted. He's a beesness man, you 'destan', an' he kan a lot o' fellers an' I vonted make him satetzfiet."

"Dot monkey?" said Jake. "Vot you talkin' aboyt! She wouldn't lishn to me neider, honesht."

"Say dot you don' vonted and dot's ull."

"Alla right; I'm goin' to ashk her, but I know it vouldn't be of naw used."

"Never min', you hask 'er foist. You knaw se wouldn't refuse you!" Joe urged, with a knowing grin.

"Hoy much vill you bet she will refushe shaw?" Jake rejoined with insincere vehemence, as he whipped out a handful of change.

"Vot kin' foon a man you are! Ulleways like to bet!" said Joe, deprecatingly. " 'F cuss it depend mit vot kin' a mout' you vill hask, you 'destan'?"

"By gum, Jaw! Vot you take me for? Ven I shay I ashk, I ashk. You knaw I don't like no monkey beeshnesh. Ven I

27

promish anytink I do it shquare, dot'sh a kin' a man *I* am!" And once more protesting his firm conviction that Mamie would disregard his request, he started to prove that she would not.

He had to traverse nearly the entire length of the hall, and, notwithstanding that he was compelled to steer clear of the dancers, he contrived to effect the passage at the swellest of his gaits, which means that he jauntily bobbed and lurched, after the manner of a blacksmith tugging at the bellows, and held up his enormous bullet head as if he were bidding defiance to the whole world. Finally he paused in front of a girl with a superabundance of pitch-black side bangs and with a pert, ill-natured, pretty face of the most strikingly Semitic cast in the whole gathering. She looked twenty-three or more, was inclined to plumpness, and her shrewd deep dark eyes gleamed out of a warm gipsy complexion. Jake found her seated in a fatigued attitude on a chair near the piano.

"Good-evenig, Mamie!" he said, bowing with mock gallantry.

"Rats!"

"Shay, Mamie, give dot feller a tvisht, vill you?"

"Dot slob again? Joe must tink if you ask me I'll get scared, ain't it? Go and tell him he is too fresh," she said with a contemptuous grimace. Like the majority of the girls of the academy, Mamie's English was a much nearer approach to a justification of its name than the gibberish spoken by the men.

Jake felt routed; but he put a bold face on it and broke out with studied resentment:

"Vot you kickin' aboyt, anyhoy? Jaw don' mean notin' at ull. If you don' vonted never min', an' dot'sh ull. It don' cut a figger, shee?" And he feignedly turned to go.

"Look how kvick he gets excited!" she said, surrenderingly.

"I ain't get ekshitet at ull; but vot'sh de used a makin' monkey beesnesh?" he retorted with triumphant acerbity.

"You are a monkey you'self," she returned with a playful pout.

The compliment was acknowledged by one of Jake's blandest grins.

"An' you are a monkey from monkeyland," he said. "Vill you dansh mit dot feller?"

28

"Rats! Vot vill you give me?"

"Vot should I give you?" he asked impatiently.

"Vill you treat?"

"Treat? Ger-rr oyt!" he replied with a sweeping kick at space.

"Den I von't dance."

"Alla right. I'll treat you mit a coupel a waltch."

"Is dot so? You must really tink I am swooning to dance vit you," she said, dividing the remark between both jargons.

"Look at her, look! she is a *regely* getzke*: one must take off one's cap to speak to her. Don't you always say you like to *dansh* with me *becush* I am a good *dansher?*"

"You must think you are a peach of a dancer, ain't it? Bennie can dance a——sight better dan you," she recurred to her English.

"Alla right!" he said tartly. "So you don' vonted?"

"O sugar! He is gettin' mad again. Vell, who is de getzke, me or you? All right, I'll dance vid de slob. But it's only becuss you ask me, mind you!" she added fawningly.

"Dot'sh alla right!" he rejoined, with an affectation of gravity, concealing his triumph. "But you makin' too much fush. I like to shpeak plain, shee? Dot'sh a kin' a man *I* am."

The next two waltzes Mamie danced with the ungainly novice, taking exaggerated pains with him. Then came a lancers, Joe calling out the successive movements huckster fashion. His command was followed by less than half of the class, however, for the greater part preferred to avail themselves of the same music for waltzing. Jake was bent upon giving Mamie what he called a "sholid good time"; and, as she shared his view that a square or fancy dance was as flimsy an affair as a stick of candy, they joined or, rather, led the seceding majority. They spun along with all-forgetful gusto; every little while he lifted her on his powerful arm and gave her a "mill," he yelping and she squeaking for sheer ecstasy, as he did so; and throughout the performance his face and his whole figure seemed to be exclaiming, "Dot'sh a kin' a man *I* am!"

Several waifs stood in a cluster admiring or begrudging the antics of the star couple. Among these was lanky Miss Jacobs

* A crucifix.

29

and Fanny the Preacher, who had shortly before made her appearance in the hall, and now stood pale and forlorn by the "apron-check" girl's side.

"Look at the way she is stickin' to him!" the little girl observed with envious venom, her gaze riveted to Mamie, whose shapely head was at this moment reclining on Jake's shoulders, with her eyes half shut, as if melting in a transport of bliss.

Fanny felt cut to the quick.

"You are jealous, ain't you?" she jerked out.

"Who, me? Vy should I be jealous?" Miss Jacobs protested, colouring. "On my part let them bo go to ——. *You* must be jealous. Here, here! See how your eyes are creeping out looking! Here, here!" she teased her offender in Yiddish, poking her little finger at her as she spoke.

"Will you shut your scurvy mouth, little piece of ugliness, you? Such a piggish apron check!" poor Fanny burst out under her breath, tears starting to her eyes.

"Such a nasty little runt!" another girl chimed in.

"Such a little cricket already knows what 'jealous' is!" a third of the bystanders put in. "You had better go home or your mamma will give you a spanking." Whereat the little cricket made a retort, which had better be left unrecorded.

"To think of a bit of a flea like that having so much *cheek!* Here is America for you!"

"America for a country and *'dod'll do'* [that'll do] for a language!" observed one of the young men of the group, indulging one of the stereotype jokes of the Ghetto.

The passage at arms drew Jake's attention to the little knot of spectators, and his eye fell on Fanny. Whereupon he summarily relinquished his partner on the floor, and advanced toward his shopmate, who, seeing him approach, hastened to retreat to the girls' bench, where she remained seated with a drooping head.

"Hello, Fanny!" he shouted briskly, coming up in front of her.

"Hello!" she returned rigidly, her eyes fixed on the dirty floor.

"Come, give ush a tvisht, vill you?"

"But you ain't goin' by Joe to-night!" she answered, with a withering curl of her lip, her glance still on the ground. "Go to your lady, she'll be mad atch you."

30

"I didn't vonted to gu here, honesht, Fanny. I o'ly come to tell Jaw shometin', an' dot'sh ull," he said guiltily.

"Why should you apologize?" she addressed the tip of her shoe in her mother tongue. "As if he was obliged to apologize to me! *For my part* you can *dance* with her day and night. *Vot do I care?* As if I *cared!* I have only come to see what a *bluffer* you are. Do you think I am a *fool?* As *smart* as your Mamie, *anyvay.* As if I had not known he wanted to make me stay at home! What are you afraid of? Am I in your way then? As if I was in his way! What business have I to be in your way? Who is in your way?"

While she was thus speaking in her voluble, querulous, harassing manner, Jake stood with his hands in his trousers' pockets, in an attitude of mock attention. Then, suddenly losing patience, he said:

"*Dot'sh alla right!* You will finish your sermon afterward. And in the meantime *lesh have a valtz* from the land of *valtzes!*" With which he forcibly dragged her off her seat, catching her round the waist.

"But I don't need it, I don't wish it! Go to your Mamie!" she protested, struggling. "I tell you I don't need it, I don't ——" The rest of the sentence was choked off by her violent breathing; for by this time she was spinning with Jake like a top. After another moment's pretense at struggling to free herself she succumbed, and presently clung to her partner, the picture of triumph and beatitude.

Meanwhile Mamie had walked up to Joe's side, and without much difficulty caused him to abandon the lancers party to themselves, and to resume with her the waltz which Jake had so abruptly broken off.

In the course of the following intermission she diplomatically seated herself beside her rival, and paraded her tranquillity of mind by accosting her with a question on shop matters. Fanny was not blind to the manœuvre, but her exultation was all the greater for it, and she participated in the ensuing conversation with exuberant geniality.

By-and-by they were joined by Jake.

"Vell, vill you treat, Jake?" said Mamie.

"Vot you vant, a kish?" he replied, putting his offer in action as well as in language.

Mamie slapped his arm.

"May the Angel of Death kiss you!" said her lips in Yiddish. "Try again!" her glowing face overruled them in a dialect of its own.

Fanny laughed.

"Once I am *treating*, both *ladas* must be *treated* alike, *ain't it?*" remarked the gallant, and again he proved himself as good as his word, although Fanny struggled with greater energy and ostensibly with more real indignation.

"But vy don't you treat, you stingy loafer you?"

"Vot elsh you vant? A peench?" He was again on the point of suiting the action to the word, but Mamie contrived to repay the pinch before she had received it, and added a generous piece of profanity into the bargain. Whereupon there ensued a scuffle of a character which defies description in more senses than one.

Nevertheless Jake marched his two "ladas" up to the marble fountain, and regaled them with two cents' worth of soda each.

An hour or so later, when Jake got out into the street, his breast pocket was loaded with a fresh batch of "Professor Peltner's Grand Annual Ball" tickets, and his two arms—with Mamie and Fanny respectively.

"As soon as I get my wages I'll call on the installment agent and give him a deposit for a steamship ticket," presently glimmered through his mind, as he adjusted his hold upon the two girls, snugly gathering them to his sides.

The Rise of David Levinsky

Jake Mindels was a devotee of Madame Klesmer, the leading Jewish actress of that period, which, by the way, was, practically the opening chapter in the interesting history of the Yiddish stage in America. Madame Klesmer was a tragedienne and a prima donna at once—a usual combination in those days.

One Friday evening we were in the gallery of her theater. The play was an "historical opera," and she was playing the part of a Biblical princess. It was the closing scene of an act. The whole company was on the stage, swaying sidewise and singing with the princess, her head in a halo of electric light in the center. Jake was feasting his large blue eyes on her. Presently he turned to me with the air of one confiding a secret. "Wouldn't you like to kiss her?" And, swinging around again, he resumed feasting his blue eyes on the princess.

"I have seen prettier women than she," I replied.

" 'S-sh! Let a fellow listen. She is a dear, all the same. You don't know a good thing when you see it, Levinsky."

"Are you in love with her?"

" 'S-sh! Do let me listen."

When the curtain fell he made me applaud her. There were several curtain-calls, during all of which he kept applauding her furiously, shouting the prima donna's name at the top of his voice and winking to me imploringly to do the same. When quiet had been restored at last I returned to the subject:

"Are you in love with her?"

A chapter from *The Rise of David Levinsky* by Abraham Cahan, published by Harper's, New York, 1917.

"Sure," he answered, without blushing. "As if a fellow could help it. If she let me kiss her little finger I should be the happiest man in the world."

"And if she let you kiss her cheek?"

"I should go crazy."

"And if she let you kiss her lips?"

"What's the use asking idle questions?"

"Would you like to kiss her neck?"

"You ask me foolish questions."

"You *are* in love with her," I declared, reflectively.

"I should say I was."

It was a unique sort of love, for he wanted me also to be in love with her.

"If you are not in love with her you must have a heart of iron, or else your soul is dry as a raisin." With which he took to analyzing the prima donna's charms, going into raptures over her eyes, smile, gestures, manner of opening her mouth, and her swing and step as she walked over the stage.

"No, I don't care for her," I replied.

"You are a peculiar fellow."

"If I did fall in love," I said, by way of meeting him half-way, "I should choose Mrs. Segalovitch. She is a thousand times prettier than Mrs. Klesmer."

"Tut, tut!"

Mrs. Segalovitch was certainly prettier than the prima donna, but she played unimportant parts, so the notion of one's falling in love with her seemed queer to Jake.

That night I had an endless chain of dreams, in every one of which Madame Klesmer was the central figure. When I awoke in the morning I fell in love with her, and was overjoyed.

When I saw Jake Mindels at dinner I said to him, with the air of one bringing glad news:

"Do you know, I *am* in love with her?"

"With whom? With Mrs. Segalovitch?"

"Oh, pshaw! I had forgotten all about her. I mean Madame Klesmer," I said, self-consciously.

Somehow, my love for the actress did not interfere with my longing thoughts of Matilda. I asked myself no questions.

And so we went on loving jointly, Jake and I, the companionship of our passion apparently stimulating our romance as companionship at a meal stimulates the appetite of the diners. Each of us seemed to be infatuated with Madame Klesmer. Yet the community of this feeling, far from arousing mutual jealousy in us, seemed to strengthen the ties of our friendship.

We would hum her songs in duet, recite her lines, compare notes on our dreams of happiness with her. One day we composed a love-letter to her, a long epistle full of Biblical and homespun poetry, which we copied jointly, his lines alternating with mine, and which we signed: "Your two lovelorn slaves whose hearts are panting for a look of your star-like eyes. Jacob and David." We mailed the letter without affixing any address.

The next evening we were in the theater, and when she appeared on the stage and shot a glance to the gallery Jake nudged me violently.

"But she does not know we are in the gallery," I argued. "She must think we are in the orchestra."

"Hearts are good guessers."

"Guessers nothing."

" 'S-sh! Let's listen."

Madame Klesmer was playing the part of a girl in a modern Russian town. She declaimed her lines, speaking like a prophetess in ancient Israel, and I liked it extremely. I was fully aware that it was unnatural for a girl in a modern Russian town to speak like a prophetess in ancient Israel, but that was just why I liked it. I thought it perfectly proper that people on the stage should not talk as they would off the stage. I thought that this unnatural speech of theirs was one of the principal things an audience paid for. The only actor who spoke like a human being was the comedian, and this, too, seemed to be perfectly proper, for a comedian was a fellow who did not take his art seriously, and so I thought that this natural talk of his was part of his fun-making. I thought it was something like a clown burlesquing the Old Testament by reading it, not in the ancient intonations of the synagogue, but in the plain, conversational accents of every-day life.

During the intermission, in the course of our talk about Madame Klesmer, Jake said:

"Do you know, Levinsky, I don't think you really love her."

"I love her as much as you, and more, too," I retorted.

"How much *do* you love her? Would you walk from New York to Philadelphia if she wanted you to do so?"

"Why should she? What good would it do her?"

"But suppose she does want it?"

"How can I suppose such nonsense?"

"Well, she might just want to see how much you love her."

"A nice test, that."

"Oh, well, she might just get that kind of notion. Women are liable to get any kind of notion, don't you know."

"Well, if Madame Klesmer got that kind of notion I should tell her to walk to Philadelphia herself."

"Then you don't love her."

"I love her as much as you do, but if she took it into her head to make a fool of me I should send her to the eighty devils."

He winced. "And you call that love, don't you?" he said, with a sneer in the corner of his pretty mouth. "As for me, I should walk to Boston, if she wanted me to."

"Even if she did not promise to let you kiss her?"

"Even if she did not."

"And if she did?"

"I should walk to Chicago."

"And if she promised to be your mistress?"

"Oh, what's the use talking that way?" he protested, blushing.

"Aren't you shy! A regular bride-to-be, I declare."

"Stop!" he said, coloring once again.

It dawned upon me that he was probably chaste, and, searching his face with a mocking look, I said:

"I bet you you are still innocent."

"Leave me alone, please," he retorted, softly.

"I have hit it, then," I importuned him, with a great sense of my own superiority.

"Do let me alone, will you?"

"I just want you to tell me whether you are innocent or not."

"It's none of your business."

"Of course you are."

"And if I am? Is it a disgrace?"

"Who says it is?"

36

I desisted. He became more attractive than ever to me.

Nevertheless, I made repeated attempts to deprave him. His chastity bothered me. The idea of breaking it down became an irresistible temptation. I would ridicule him for a sissy, appeal to him in the name of his health, beg him as one does for a personal favor, all in vain.

He spoke better English than I, with more ease, and in that pretty basso of his which I envied. He had never read Dickens or any other English author, but he was familiar with some subjects to which I was a stranger. He was well grounded in arithmetic, knew some geography, and now with a view of qualifying for the study of medicine, he was preparing, with the aid of a private teacher, for the Regents' examination in algebra, geometry, English composition, American and English history. I thought he did not study "deeply" enough, that he took more real interest in his collars and neckties, the shine of his shoes, or the hang of his trousers than he did in his algebra or history.

By his cleanliness and tidiness he reminded me of Naphtali, which, indeed, had something to do with my attachment for him. My relations toward him echoed with the feelings I used to have for the reticent, omniscient boy of Abner's Court, and with the hoarse, studious young Talmudist with whom I would "famish in company." He had neither Naphtali's brains nor his individuality, yet I looked up to him and was somewhat under his influence. I adopted many of the English phrases he was in the habit of using and tried to imitate his way of dressing. As a consequence, he would sometimes assume a patronizing tone with me, addressing me with a good-natured sneer which I liked in spite of myself.

We made a compact to speak nothing but English, and, to a considerable extent, we kept it.

37

MORRIS RAPHAEL COHEN

The philosopher Morris Raphael Cohen was born in Minsk, Russia, in 1880, the son of Abraham Cohen and Bessie (Farfel) Cohen. His maternal grandfather, who supervised his earliest education, made a tremendous and lifelong impression upon him, and one feels at times that he subjected all his later successes and experiences in life to critical skepticism suggested by the standards of judgment learned from his grandfather (who was, of course, a very rigid Orthodox Jew, anything but a skeptic).

Against this grandfather's wishes and better judgment and against his own wishes at the time, too, little Morris was brought to the United States at the age of twelve. He went through elementary and high school in three years, winning a gold medal for excellence in mathematics on graduation. His grandfather, in the old country, informed of this triumph by his brilliant grandson, commented briefly and bitterly: "Gold does not change its nature, unlike yourself." (He was aware, it seems, that the young man was even then falling away from Orthodox ritual.) He entered the College of the City of New York, from which he was to receive his B.S. degree in 1900 and with which he was to be associated for the greater part of his remaining life. In 1906, he received his Ph.D. degree from Harvard with high commendations from his great and famous teachers there: William James and Josiah Royce.

From 1899 to 1907 he taught at the Educational Alliance and at the Davidson Collegiate Institute as well. He taught at his alma mater, C.C.N.Y., from 1902 until his retirement in 1938. In his early years there, he taught mathematics; later on, of course, he

39

became associated with the Department of Philosophy, which in his time included, in addition to himself, the nationally well-known lecturer and writer Harry Alan Overstreet, who served as Chairman and befriended Cohen and saved him from the administrative tasks which might otherwise have devolved upon him. In Cohen's time, teaching at the City College involved an inordinately heavy teaching load, and this was probably responsible for his relatively early retirement from his duties there in 1938. After his retirement, he served as Professor of Philosophy at the University of Chicago.

The students at C.C.N.Y., who were not too awe-struck by his reputation with such men as Bertrand Russell and John Dewey to speak up freely to him, stimulated him very much, according to his own testimony. Most of them regarded him with awe as a "modern Socrates with an acid tongue." He lectured at various times at Harvard, Yale, Columbia, Johns Hopkins, Stanford, St. Johns, and the New School for Social Research.

He married Mary Ryshpan in 1906, and among his children was the eminent legal philosopher Felix Cohen, who helped to edit some of his father's works after his death. Morris Cohen served as President of the American Philosophical Association in 1929 and on the council of the American Association of University Professors from 1918 to 1921. He was a Fellow of the American Association for the Advancement of Science and organized the Conference on Jewish Relations in 1933.

Harold Laski once called Cohen "the most penetrating and creative U.S. philosopher since William James," and Sidney Hook, one of his own pupils, said he embodied "the spirit of intelligent dissent" and held "the foremost place in the realm of creative American thought" of his day. Cohen was the editor of the Modern Legal Philosophy series and of *Jewish Social Studies*. He contributed a major article to the *Cambridge History of American Literature* and contributed to *Contemporary American Philosophy*.

He died on January 28, 1947, and a great many of his most important publications were posthumous. During his lifetime, his major work was entitled *Reason and Nature*. His posthumous and unfinished autobiography, *A Dreamer's Journey* (edited by his son Felix), was described by Felix Frankfurter (a fellow

40

student during his years at Harvard) as "an effort, and a triumphal one, as was Morris Cohen's whole life, after things that are of perennial value." Perry Miller in the *Nation* said of it: "It will demand a permanent place among the classics of immigrant narrative and one not too far behind the greater classics of intellectual biography." The well-known popularizer of semantics, S. I. Hayakawa, attributed to Cohen "that combination of learning and ethical earnestness and sweetness of temper that Matthew Arnold called 'urbanity.' "

It is perhaps a general rule that the best and most lasting literary accounts of any given time do not emerge until long afterward. Even when contemporary events are recorded immediately, so long as the recording is not journalism aimed in the direction of the immediate present but is meant to be withheld from publication until a more or less remote future, there is something imponderable that accrues to the author and his work. Call the quality disinterestedness, proportion, measure, what you will, it is unmistakably there, and though it is by itself not a sufficient guarantee of immortality it appears to be a condition of it. Pepys' *Diary*, Saint-Simon's *Memoirs*, Boswell's *Journals*, Rousseau's *Confessions*, Madame de Sévigné's *Letters*—all without exception appeared after their authors' death, and the list of distinguished works concerning which this is true might be almost indefinitely extended from ancient literature to the most contemporary, from Petronius' *Satyricon* to Eugene O'Neill's *Long Day's Journey into Night*. And not only works whose vertebrae consist of facts but those that are fictional as well become enriched, like old wine, with the passage of time.

"The sunshine of the light of letters," wrote Whitman in his famous Preface of 1855, "is simplicity. Nothing is better than simplicity!" Cohen's autobiography (another in the long list of distinguished posthumous works) is one that illustrates the validity of this aphorism. Despite its profundity, the clarity of its analysis places no needless obstacles between less developed intellectual understandings and its own. The book speaks in plain words about basic and universal subjects of human interest and concern. Many people, who do not know it or know no more of it than its name or the name of its author, are capable, it seems to me, both of enjoying and learning from *A Dreamer's Journey*.

41

A Dreamer's Journey

The life of the East Side in the days of my adolescence was characterized by a feverish intensity of intellectual life and a peculiar restlessness. We had no patience with the prevailing evils and corruptions of the day. Our eagerness to help usher in a better social order was well-nigh desperate and our anxiety about our own achievements and shortcomings in this endeavor was almost morbid. In all this we reflected not only the traditional current of European Jewish life, with its emphasis upon intellectual values, but also the impact of the New World on eyes that could see its problems and potentialities with the fresh vision generally ascribed to foreign visitors or to the "man from Mars."

The eastern Jewish immigrants to this country in the 1890's had, for the most part, been subjected to a highly rigorous training along pietistic lines. Ten hours or more of study day after day took up the childhood of every self-respecting eastern Jewish boy. Fortunate were those who were permitted to continue this routine as students of the Talmud, as teachers or as rabbis for the rest of their lives. Those not so fortunate were expected to devote the same long hours and endless energies to the mastering of some trade or business. But even those who were not permitted to devote their adult years primarily to learning were expected to devote a considerable portion of their time to reading, prayer, and argument, carried on in a sacred language and dealing largely with a totally foreign environment.

The migration to the New World broke the old patterns. The old limitations on the proper subjects of intellectual inquiry and

Selection from *A Dreamer's Journey* by Morris Raphael Cohen, published simultaneously by Beacon Press, Boston, and The Free Press, Glencoe, Ill., 1949.

discussion were removed, but the intellectual passion, the tradition of study, the high value which the family circle put upon learning and skill continued. Parents continued to grind their own lives to the bone in order to make it possible for their children to achieve some intellectual distinction or skill that might be considered a New World substitute for the Talmudic learning which represented the highest achievement in the old environment. So it was that many of the first generation and many more of the second, despite the difficulties of a new environment and a strange language, brought to the tasks which the New World presented a force that was more than the force of any single individual. It was as if a great dam had broken and the force of water accumulated over many years had been let loose. This mighty force permeated every nook and corner of human endeavor.

Opinions may differ as to the worth of many of the enterprises to which this force was directed. The second generation had its boxers, gamblers and shyster lawyers, as well as great judges, teachers and scientists. Doctors, movie magnates, writers, merchants, philanthropists, communists or defenders of corporate wealth all showed an intensity that must have seemed a bit outlandish to the more comfortable and easy-going segments of the American population. Perhaps something of the same intensity characterized earlier American generations disciplined under the hard patterns of Puritan, Quaker or Mormon protests against the life of ease and comfort.

This intensity of life, this striving for perfection in diverse fields, surrounded me and the men and women of my generation at the turn of the century, in City College and in the various clubs, circles and societies that dotted our intellectual horizons.

The habit of organizing groups of kindred spirits about some teacher or moral leader, for the purpose of solving the world's problems, goes very far back in the Hebraic tradition. The spirit that infused our various groups and societies was expressed with particular clarity in a letter of Thomas Davidson's:

> There is nothing that the world of to-day needs so much as a new order of social relations, a new feeling between man and man. We may talk and teach as long as we like, but until we have a new so-

ciety with ideal relations and aims we have accomplished very little. All great world movements begin with a little knot of people, who, in their individual lives, and in their relations to each other, realize the ideal that is to be. To live truth is better than to utter it. Isaiah would have prophesied in vain, had he not gathered round him a little band of disciples who lived according to his ideal. . . . Again, what would the teachings of Jesus have amounted to had he not collected a body of disciples, who made it their life-aim to put his teachings into practice. . . .

You will perhaps think I am laying out a mighty task for you, a task far above your powers and aspirations; but it is not so. Every great change in individual and social conditions—and we are on the verge of such a change—begins small, among simple earnest people, face to face with the facts of life. Ask yourselves seriously, "Why should not the coming change begin with us?" And you will find that there is no reason why the new world, the world of righteousness, kindliness and enlightenment for which we are all longing and toiling, may not date from us as well as from anybody. A little knot of earnest Jews has turned the world upside down before now. Why may not the same thing—nay a far better thing—happen in your day and among you? Have you forgotten the old promise made to Abraham: "In thy seed shall all the nations of the earth be blessed"?

This was the spirit in which, even before Davidson came among us, we organized in our literary, socialist, and philosophical clubs and circles. After the demise of the Bryant Literary Society, in the summer of 1896, I became involved for a year or so in another literary society beginning in the spring of 1897. This we called the Young Men's Literary Society. Among its members were Louis Lande, Rosen, Dave Klein, Friedman, Leo Jacobs, Schiff, Ben Ridgik, Shlivek and Rosenblatt, our leader and critic. Mr. Isaac Spectorsky, the Superintendent of the Educational Alliance, was also interested in the Comte Synthetic Circle, an organization led by Edward King. He proposed that our Young Men's Literary Society should join the latter organization. The move was not popular, but I was the only one who had the courage (or lack of chivalry) to voice an objection, and my objection prevailed. This was, of course, before I met Mary Ryshpan and her two sisters, Bertha and Sarah, who were members of the Comte Synthetic Circle and who, along with Leonora O'Reilly, an ardent Irish Republican and a founder of the Women's Trade Union League, were its most active sponsors.

The public meetings of our Young Men's Literary Society, and my activities as editor of its journal were not marked by enthusiasm for Mark Hanna and the Republican Party, which had just succeeded in electing McKinley President. The Bryan campaign in the summer and autumn of 1896 had brought me face to face with the issues of American politics. I had been interested in the socialist movement, perhaps because the Jewish Socialist weekly, *Die Arbeiter Zeitung,* was the most intelligent newspaper that I could find. Bryan, though not a socialist, appeared to me as a great liberating force, especially after McKinley became President in the spring of 1897. During the winter of 1896–97, I helped to run a young workingmen's class on Market Street as part of my work in Daniel de Leon's Socialist Labor Party. During the election campaign of 1897, when Henry George was running for Mayor of New York, I was active in the campaign of Daniel de Leon, who was running for assemblyman in the district in which I lived. Our hopes that he might become the first Socialist representative in the New York State Legislature were not realized. On election night, I met Eugene Schoen and we decided to organize a Marx Circle. Louis Roth, Willie Hirsch, Harry Simmons, Abe Kovar, Frank Silverman, Simon Frucht, Sidney Bernstein, Jimmie Alman, Abramson (our first "editor"), and a few other congenial friends met at the Henry Street Settlement and various other meeting places to read and argue about Marx's *Das Kapital, Merrie England* and other socialist classics.

Though I had opposed joining with the Comte Synthetic Circle, I soon found myself irresistibly drawn to it. This society was organized around the personality of Edward King, whose lecture on Mill had so impressed me. I attended a good many of its meetings during the year 1898, and it was there that I came to know one whose aspirations and hopes were so close to mine that we soon became companions for life.

Mary Ryshpan was in the forefront of the struggle of those who, growing to young womanhood amidst the intellectual currents of the immigrant East Side, helped to break the Jewish tradition that had excluded women from full participation in the highest intellectual pursuits. Throughout her life she was an ardent admirer of George Eliot, whom she took as her model of womanly courage. Completely selfless in her relations with others for whom she sought to make real the opportunities of the New World, she was a teacher, guide and protector to a host of relatives and friends. In those days it was not usual for Jewish girls to go to college, and she saw to it that her advantage in this respect did not remain a personal one but was shared with all for whom she could help to open the gates of a wider and richer intellectual world.

This indestructible urge which she and I and so many of our mutual friends had, to possess for ourselves the fruits of the Age of Reason, dominated all our activities. Even in the field of social reform our socialism was, above all, not a seeking for better food or drink or clothing or even homes for ourselves and our less fortunate fellows. It was a protest against economic conditions which denied to so many of us, and to our less fortunate brothers and sisters, access to the riches of the spirit. Those who toiled twelve hours a day, month after month, from childhood to old age, were deprived of all the things that made human life worth living. And so our socialist activity, though often cast in Marx's materialistic terms, was directed primarily to the conquest and democratization of the things of the spirit.

The world that we faced on the East Side at the turn of the century presented a series of heartbreaking dilemmas. To the extent that we made the world of science and enlightenment a part of ourselves, we were inevitably torn from the traditions of narrow Orthodoxy. For some two thousand years our people had clung to their faith under the pressure of continual persecution. But now, for us at least, the walls of the ghetto had been removed. We learned that all non-Jews were not mere soulless heathens. We found that the Jews had not been the only conservators of wisdom and civilization. And having been immersed in the literature of science we called upon the old religion to justify itself on the basis of modern science and culture. But the old generation was not in a position to say how this could be done. With all respect for our old Orthodoxy, it would not be

46

honest to deny that it harbored a great deal of superstition—indeed, who is free from superstition? But because this superstition was regarded as an integral part of Judaism, because no distinction was drawn between ritual and religious convictions and feelings, the very word "religion" came to be discredited by many liberal people—who, whatever might be said about their errors, at least attempted to think for themselves.

What ensued was a struggle between the old and new ideals, resulting in a conflict between the older and younger generations fraught with heart-rending consequences. Homes ceased to be places of peace and in the ensuing discord much of the proverbial strength of the Jewish family was lost. As the home ceased to be the center of interest, the unity of life, nurtured by pride in the achievements of one's forebears and by parental pride in the achievements of children, was broken. There was scarcely a Jewish home on the East Side that was free from this friction between parents and children. This explosive tension made it possible for the same family to produce saints and sinners, philosophers and gunmen.

We might, if we could, mask our unorthodox ideas, and use the word "God," with Spinoza, to mean what scientists call the system of nature, or, by proper verbal camouflage, otherwise conceal our departures from the old, pious outlook upon the universe. Every impulse of filial piety, of gratitude to the parents who had made it possible for us to enjoy the fruits of the world of science, drove us to this hypocrisy. But to the extent that we succumbed, we could not preserve the integrity of the intellect and the spirit. And this meant that young men and women were forced to play the hypocrite at the very dawn of their moral sense. No wonder that the development of religious sentiment was stunted among us and that cynicism or pessimism came so often to displace the natural idealism of youth.

However we resolved this dilemma, and whatever concessions we made to the old ritual, the loss of the religious faith which had sustained our parents through so many generations of suffering left a void in our lives which we tried with every fiber of our beings to fill in one way or another. All our organizations and circles were attempts to fill this void. None of these attempts amounted to very much in the long run until the advent among us of a wandering Scottish philosopher [Thomas Davidson] who had been the spiritual inspiration, in England, of the Fellowship of the New Life and its more activist offshoot, the Fabian Society, as well as one of the founders of the Aristotelian Society, and who was destined to give to many of us on the East Side the same kind of inspiration that he had given to men and women like Havelock Ellis, Sidney and Beatrice Webb, and Edward Carpenter.

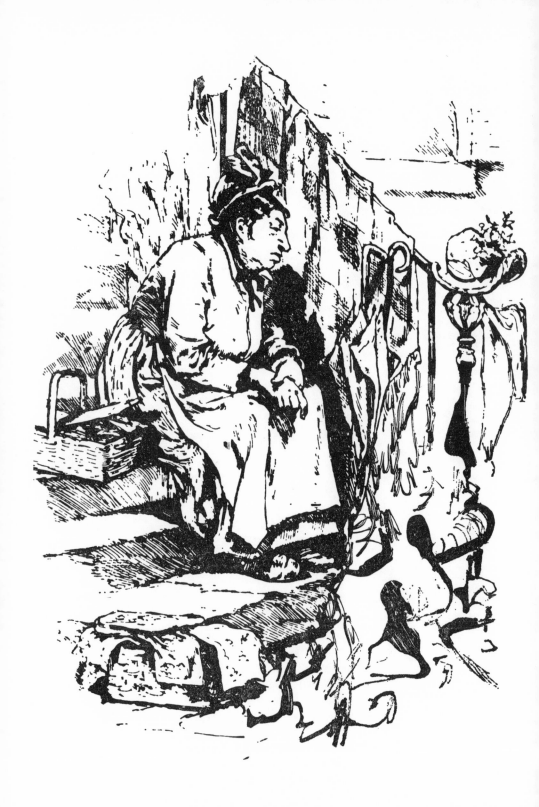

WILLIAM DEAN HOWELLS

William Dean Howells is one of the most *strategically* important figures in the history of American literature. His influence was exercised not only through his immense productivity in both journalism and literature (his long life which stretched from 1837 to 1920 produced, according to Carl Van Doren, a corresponding harvest of "fourscore books") but also through the importance of the editorial posts which he occupied, particularly at the *Atlantic Monthly* and at *Harper's Magazine,* through his eminent friendships with such diverse figures as Henry James and Mark Twain, through his generous discovery and encouragement of such talents as those of Stephen Crane, Hamlin Garland, Frank Norris, Abraham Cahan and others, and through his self-conscious championing of the new principles of literary realism in America and his polemical zeal against the romantic sentimentality so perennially popular in American fiction. Mark Twain, a great stylist himself, paid him the tribute of saying that while other writers, including himself, sometimes found the right word, Howells always found it.

He was born in a small town in Ohio, Martin's Ferry, the son of a printer-journalist, in whose office Howells learned to be a typesetter as well as a writer. He expressed pride in the fact, during his later years, that his father had built the house in which he was born "with his own capable hands." He worked for a number of newspapers while he was growing up, as reporter, editor and typesetter. Here he got most of his education, becoming well-read in authors of several modern tongues and schooling himself in the effective use of the English language. In 1860, he

51

had made his mark sufficiently as both writer and editor of an important Republican newspaper to be given the job of writing the campaign biography of Lincoln. For his services, after the crucial election, he was named Consul to Venice and spent the years of the Civil War abroad. On his return in 1865, he was a writer for the *Tribune* and the *Nation* in New York and in 1871 went to Boston as assistant editor of the *Atlantic,* becoming editor in the following year when he was thirty-five years old. In addition to his editorial tasks, he served as lecturer at Harvard and fitted comfortably into the rarefied New England intellectual atmosphere. Much earlier, there had been an indication of his acceptance at the highest levels in a note which Hawthorne had written to Emerson saying, "I find this young man worthy."

It is generally agreed by literary historians that Howells' move from Boston to New York in 1885 marked more than the end of an epoch and the beginning of another in his own life. It also marked a transition in the culture of the country as a whole when dominance definitely passed from the center of New England two hundred miles south to the great cosmopolitan megalopolis. The world in which he now lived was so different from the one he left that he could say: "Boston seems of another planet." Europe had meant a lot to Howells ever since he had lived there and probably before, but its power over him (not, of course, to the point of tempting him to become an expatriate like his friend Henry James) increased while he lived in the American city which in many ways is closer to Europe than any other. His affinity for the naturalistic novel of Zola (so far as taste was concerned rather than practice) and the greater Russians like Tolstoy became interlaced with concern about economics, politics, and the social question in general.

His admiration and sympathy for Russian Jewish socialists like Abraham Cahan must be understood in the context of his sympathy for the working class in general, which was shown by various statements on labor questions (such as the New York streetcar strike) and by the novels he wrote in the 1890's. His creative works of this period are described by scholars as bordering upon tracts. In this sense, his development for a time reversed that which we can observe in a man like Cahan. The latter was striving to free himself from the demands of journalism and propaganda and to enter the freer world of imaginative creation, while Howells was finding the comedies of manners as they unfolded in ordinary middle-class American life, at which he excelled and which constitute his lasting contribution to American literature, less and less of a satisfaction and fulfillment for himself as a conscientious social being.

Yet he never became alienated from the mainstream of his country's life and its assumptions, as Henry James so demonstratively did or as Mark Twain did more secretively and privately. It was not merely a play on his middle name that was responsible for his being known for many years as "the Dean of American letters." He was the first President of the American Academy of Arts and Letters and received the Gold Medal from the National Institute. He was honored by degrees from Oxford, Yale, Harvard, Princeton, and Columbia.

In his later years and especially in those following his death, Howells came to be looked upon as a drag by the very movement which he had helped to launch many years ago. He was out of sympathy with Dreiser and lost touch even with disciples like Cahan when the latter showed in *Levinsky* that he had chosen Dreiser as his model in preference to Howells. Howells' correspondence reveals that he did not recognize any progress in Cahan's work from *Yekl*, which he approved, to *Levinsky*, of which he was much more critical. In this he was no doubt wrong. But he hardly deserved the epithets (like timid, polite, and inhibited) which it became fashionable to use in describing him.

More recently still, there have been signs that a better balanced view and appreciation of his position both historically and aesthetically will eventually prevail. Whether or not Frost's high estimate of him as one of the eight or so greatest writers that America has produced so far will be universally received, we cannot tell, but it seems safe to predict that the ultimate judgment may be somewhat closer to this evaluation than to the small-minded contempt and neglect which for a time was the rule in sophisticated circles so far as he was concerned and in reaction against which Frost perhaps spoke.

Impressions and Experiences

I do not know whether the Hebrew quarter, when I began to make my calls there, seemed any worse than the American quarter or not. But I noticed presently a curious subjective effect in myself, which I offer for the reader's speculation.

There is something in a very little experience of such places that blunts the perception, so that they do not seem so dreadful as they are; and I should feel as if I were exaggerating if I recorded my first impression of their loathsomeness. I soon came to look upon the conditions as normal, not for me, indeed, or for the kind of people I mostly consort with, but for the inmates of the dens and lairs about me. Perhaps this was partly their fault; they were uncomplaining, if not patient, in circumstances where I believe a single week's sojourn, with no more hope of a better lot than they could have, would make anarchists of the best people in the city. Perhaps the poor people themselves are not so thoroughly persuaded that there is anything very unjust in their fate, as the compassionate think. They at least do not know the better fortune of others, and they have the habit of passively enduring their own. I found them usually cheerful in the Hebrew quarter, and they had so much courage as enabled them to keep themselves noticeably clean in an environment where I am afraid their betters would scarcely have had heart to wash their faces and comb their hair. There was even a decent tidiness in their dress, which I did not find very ragged, though it often seemed unseasonable and insufficient. But here again, as in many other

Selections from William Dean Howells' *Impressions and Experiences*, published by Harper's, New York, 1896.

phases of life, I was struck by men's heroic superiority to their fate, if their fate is hard; and I felt anew that if prosperous and comfortable people were as good in proportion to their fortune as these people were they would be as the angels of light, which I am afraid they now but faintly resemble.

One of the places we visited was a court somewhat like that we had already seen in the American quarter, but rather smaller and with more the effect of a pit, since the walls around it were so much higher. There was the same row of closets at one side and the hydrant next them, but here the hydrant was bound up in rags to keep it from freezing, apparently, and the wretched place was by no means so foul under foot. To be sure, there was no stable to contribute its filth, but we learned that a suitable stench was not wanting from a bakery in one of the basements, which a man in good clothes and a large watch-chain told us rose from it in suffocating fumes at a certain hour, when the baker was doing some unimaginable thing to the bread. This man seemed to be the employer of labor in one of the rooms above, and he said that when the smell began they could hardly breathe. He caught promptly at the notion of the Board of Health, and I dare say that the baker will be duly abated. None of the other people complained, but that was perhaps because they had only their Yiddish to complain in, and knew that it would be wasted on us. They seemed neither curious nor suspicious concerning us; they let us go everywhere, as if they had no thought of hindering us. One of the tenements we entered had just been vacated; but there was a little girl of ten there, with some much smaller children, amusing them in the empty space. Through a public-spirited boy, who had taken charge of us from the beginning and had a justly humorous sense of the situation, we learned that this little maid was not the sister but the servant of the others, for even in these low levels society makes its distinctions. I dare say that the servant was not suffered to eat with the others when they had anything to eat, and that when they had nothing her inferiority was somehow brought home to her. She may have been made to wait and famish after the others had hungered some time. She was a cheerful and friendly creature and her small brood were kept tidy like herself.

55

The basement under this vacant tenement we found inhabited, and though it was a most preposterous place for people to live, it was not as dirty as one would think. To be sure, it was not very light and all the dirt may not have been visible. One of the smiling women who were there made their excuses, "Poor people; cannot keep very nice," and laughed as if she had said a good thing. There was nothing in the room but a table and a few chairs and a stove, without fire, but they were all contentedly there together in the dark, which hardly let them see one another's faces. My companion struck a match and held it to the cavernous mouth of an inner cellar half as large as the room we were in, where it winked and paled so soon that I had only a glimpse of the bed, with the rounded heap of bedding on it; but out of this hole, as if she had been a rat, scared from it by the light, a young girl came, rubbing her eyes and vaguely smiling, and vanished upstairs somewhere.

I found no shape or size of tenement but this. There was always the one room, where the inmates lived by day, and the one den, where they slept by night, apparently all in the same bed, though probably the children were strewn about the floor. If the tenement were high up the living-room had more light and air than if it were low down; but the sleeping-hole never had any light or air of its own. My calls were made on one of the mild days which fell before last Christmas, and so I suppose I saw these places at their best; but what they must be when the summer is seven times heated without, as it often is in New York, or when the arctic cold has pierced these hapless abodes and the inmates huddle together for their animal heat, the reader must imagine for himself. The Irish-Americans had flaming stoves, even on that soft day, but in the Hebrew tenements I found no fire. They were doubtless the better for this, and it is one of the comical anomalies of the whole affair that they are singularly healthy. The death rate among them is one of the lowest in the city, though whether for their final advantage it might not better be the highest, is one of the things one must not ask one's self. In their presence I should not dare to ask it, even in my deepest thought. They are then so like other human beings and really so little different from the best, except in their environment, that I had to get away from this before I could regard them as wild beasts.

I suppose there are and have been worse conditions of life, but if I stopped short of savage life I found it hard to imagine them. I did not exaggerate to myself the squalor that I saw, and I do not exaggerate it to the reader. As I have said, I was so far from sentimentalizing it that I almost immediately reconciled myself to it, as far as its victims were concerned. Still, it was squalor of a kind which, it seemed to me, it could not be possible to outrival anywhere in the life one commonly calls civilized. It is true that the Indians who formerly inhabited this island were no more comfortably lodged in their wigwams of bark and skins than these poor New Yorkers in their tenements. But the wild men pay no rent, and if they are crowded together upon terms that equally forbid decency and comfort in their shelter, they have the freedom of the forest and the prairie about them; they have the illimitable sky and the whole light of day and the four winds to breathe when they issue into the open air. The New York tenement dwellers, even when they leave their lairs, are still pent in their high-walled streets, and inhale a thousand stenches of their own and others' making. The street, except in snow and rain, is always better than their horrible houses, and it is doubtless because they pass so much of their time in the street that the death rate is so low among them. Perhaps their domiciles can be best likened for darkness and discomfort to the dugouts or sod huts of the settlers on the great plains. But these are only temporary shelters, while the tenement dwellers have no hope of better housing; they have neither the prospect of a happier fortune through their own energy as the settlers have, nor any chance from the humane efforts and teachings of missionaries, like the savages. With the tenement dwellers it is from generation to generation, if not for the individual, then for the class, since no one expects that there will not always be tenement dwellers in New York as long as our present economical conditions endure.

When I first set out on my calls I provided myself with some small silver, which I thought I might fitly give, at least to the children, and in some of the first places I did this. But presently I began to fancy an unseemliness in it, as if it were an indignity added to the hardship of their lot, and to feel that unless I gave all my worldly wealth to them I was in a manner mocking their misery. I could not give everything, for then I should have had to come upon charity myself, and so I mostly kept my little coins in my pocket; but when we mounted into the court again from that cellar apartment and found an old, old woman there, wrinkled and yellow, with twinkling eyes and a toothless smile, waiting to see us, as if she were as curious in her way as we were in ours, I was tempted. She said in her Yiddish, which the humorous boy interpreted, that she was eighty years old, and she looked a hundred, while she babbled unintelligibly but very cheerfully on. I gave her a piece of twenty-five cents and she burst into a blessing, that I should not have thought could be bought for money. We did not stay to hear it out, but the boy did, and he followed to report it to me, with a gleeful interest in its beneficent exaggerations. If it is fulfilled I shall live to be a man of many and prosperous years, and I shall die possessed of wealth that will endow a great many colleges and found a score of libraries. I do not know whether the boy envied me or not, but I wish I could have left that benediction to him, for I took a great liking to him, his shrewd smile, his gay eyes, his promise of a Hebrew nose, and his whole wise little visage. He said that he went to school and studied reading, writing, geography and everything. All the children we spoke to said that they went to school, and they were quick and intelligent. They could mostly speak English, while most of their elders knew only Yiddish.

The sound of this was around us on the street we issued into, and which seemed from end to end a vast bazaar, where there was a great deal of selling, whether there was much buying or not. The place is humorously called the pig-market by the Christians, because everything in the world but pork is to be found there. To me its activity was a sorrowfully amusing satire upon the business ideal of our plutocratic civilization. These people were desperately poor, yet they preyed upon one another in the commerce, as if they could be enriched by selling dear or buying cheap. So far as I could see they would only impoverish each other more and more, but they trafficked as eagerly as if there were wealth in every bargain. The sidewalks and the roadways were thronged with peddlers and purchasers, and everywhere I saw splendid types of that old Hebrew world which had the sense if not the knowledge of God when all the rest of us lay sunk in heathen darkness. There were women with oval faces and olive tints, and clear, dark eyes, relucent as evening pools, and men with long beards of jetty black or silvery white, and the noble profiles of their race. I said to myself that it was among such throngs that Christ walked, it was from such people that he chose his Disciples and his friends; but I looked in vain for him in Hester Street. Probably he was at that moment in Fifth Avenue.

After all, I was loath to come away. I should have liked to stay and live awhile with such as they, if the terms of their life had been possible, for there were phases of it that were very attractive. That constant meeting and that neighborly intimacy were superficially at least of a very pleasant effect, and though the whole place seemed abandoned to mere trade, it may have been a necessity of the case, for I am told that many of these Hebrews have another ideal, and think and vote in the hope that the land of their refuge shall yet some day keep its word to the world, so that men shall be equally free in it to the pursuit of happiness. I suppose they are mostly fugitives from the Russian persecution, and that from the cradle their days must have been full of fear and care, and from the time they could toil that they must have toiled at whatever their hands found to do. Yet they had not the look of a degraded people; they were quiet and orderly, and I saw none of the drunkenness or the truculence of an Irish or low American neighborhood among them. There were no policemen in sight, and the quiet behavior that struck me so much seemed not to have been enforced. Very likely they may have moods different from that I saw, but I only tell of what I saw, and I am by no means ready yet to preach poverty as a saving grace. Though they seemed so patient and even cheerful in some cases, I do not think it is well for human beings to live whole families together in one room with a kennel out of it, where modesty may survive, but decency is impossible. Neither do I think they can be the better men and women for being insufficiently clothed and fed, though so many of us appear none the better for being housed in palaces and clad in purple and fine linen and faring sumptuously every day.

I have tried to report simply and honestly what I saw of the

59

life of our poorest people that day. One might say it was not so bad as it is painted, but I think it is quite as bad as it appeared; and I could not see that in itself or in its conditions it held the promise or the hope of anything better. If it is tolerable, it must endure; if it is intolerable, still it must endure. Here and there one will release himself from it, and doubtless numbers are always doing this, as in the days of slavery there were always fugitives; but for the great mass the captivity remains. Upon the present terms of leaving the poor to be housed by private landlords, whose interest it is to get the greatest return of money for the money invested, the very poorest must always be housed as they are now. Nothing but public control in some form or other can secure them a shelter fit for human beings.

When I come home from these walks of mine, I have a vision of the wretched quarters through which I have passed, as blotches of disease upon the civic body, as loathsome sores, destined to eat deeper and deeper into it; and I am haunted by this sense of them, until I plunge deep into the Park, and wash my consciousness clean of it all for a while. But when I am actually in these leprous spots, I become hardened, for the moment, to the deeply underlying fact of human discomfort. I feel their picturesqueness, with a callous indifference to that ruin, or that defect, which must so largely constitute the charm of the picturesque. A street of tenement-houses is always more picturesque than a street of brownstone residences, which the same thoroughfare usually is before it slopes to either river. The fronts of the edifices are decorated with the iron balconies and ladders of the fire-escapes, and have in the perspective a false air of gayety, which is travestied in their rear by the lines thickly woven from the windows to the tall poles set between the backs of the houses, and fluttering with drying clothes as with banners.

The sidewalks swarm with children, and the air rings with their clamor, as they fly back and forth at play; on the thresholds, the mothers sit nursing their babes, and the old women gossip together; young girls lean from the casements, alow and aloft, or flirt from the doorways with the hucksters who leave their carts in the street, while they come forward with some bargain in fruit or vegetables, and then resume their leisurely progress and their jarring cries. The place has all the attraction of close neighborhood, which the poor love, and which affords them for nothing the spectacle of the human drama, with themselves for actors. In a picture it would be most pleasingly effective, for then you could be in it, and yet have the distance on it which it needs. But to be in it, and not have the distance, is to inhale the stenches of the neglected street, and to catch that yet fouler and dreadfuller poverty-smell which breathes from the open doorways. It is to see the children quarrelling in their games, and beating each other in the face, and rolling each other in the gutter, like the little savage outlaws they are. It is to see the work-worn look of the mothers, the squalor of the babes, the haggish ugliness of the old women, the slovenly frowziness of the young girls. All this makes you hasten your pace down to the river, where the tall buildings break and dwindle into stables and shanties of wood, and finally end in the piers, commanding the whole stretch of the mighty waterway with its shipping, and the wooded heights of its western bank.

I am supposing you to have walked down a street of tenement houses to the North River, as the New Yorkers call the Hudson; and I wish I could give some notion of the beauty and majesty of the stream, some sense of the mean and ignoble effect of the city's invasion of the hither shore. The ugliness is, indeed, only worse in degree, but not in kind, than that of all city water-fronts. Instead of pleasant homes, with green lawns and orchards sloping to the brink, huge factories and foundries, lumber yards, breweries, slaughter-houses, and warehouses, abruptly interspersed with stables and hovels and drinking-saloons, disfigure the shore, and in the nearest avenue the freight trains come and go on lines of railroads, in all the middle portion of New York. South of it, in the business section, the poverty section, the river region is a mere chaos of industrial and commercial strife and pauper wretchedness. North of it there are gardened drive-ways following the shore; and even at many points between, when you finally reach the river, there is a kind of peace, or at least a truce to the frantic activities of business. To be sure, the heavy trucks grind up and down the long piers, but on either side the docks are

61

full of leisurely canal-boats, and if you could come with me in the late afternoon, you would see the smoke curling upward from their cabin roofs, as from the chimneys of so many rustic cottages, and smell the evening meal cooking within, while the canal-wives lounged at the gangway hatches for a breath of the sunset air, and the boatmen smoked on the gunwales or indolently plied the long sweeps of their pumps. All the hurry and turmoil of the city is lost among these people, whose clumsy craft recall the grassy inland levels remote from the metropolis, and the slow movement of life in the quiet country ways. Some of the mothers from the tenement-houses stroll down on the piers with their babies in their arms, and watch their men-kind, of all ages, fishing along the sides of the dock, or casting their lines far out into the current at the end. They do not seem to catch many fish, and never large ones, but they silently enjoy the sport, which they probably find leisure for in the general want of work in these hard times; if they swear a little at their luck, now and then, it is, perhaps, no more than their luck deserves. Some do not even fish, but sit with their legs dangling over the water, and watch the swift tugs, or the lagging sloops that pass, with now and then a larger sail, or a towering passenger steamboat. Far down the stream they can see the forests of masts, fringing either shore, and following the point of the island round and up into the great channel called the East River. These vessels seem as multitudinous as the houses that spread everywhere from them over the shore farther than the eye can reach. They bring the commerce of the world to this mighty city, which, with all its riches, is the parent of such misery, and with all its traffic abounds in idle men who cannot find work. The ships look happy and free, in the stream, but they are of the overworked world, too, as well as the houses; and let them spread their wings ever so widely, they still bear with them the sorrows of the poor.

The other evening I walked over to the East River through one of the tenement streets, and I reached the waterside just as the soft night was beginning to fall in all its autumnal beauty. The afterglow died from the river, while I hung upon a parapet over a gulf ravined out of the bank for a street, and experienced that artistic delight which cultivated people are often proud of feeling, in the aspect of the long prison island which breaks the expanse of the channel. I knew the buildings on it were prisons, and that the men and women in them, bad before, could only come out of them worse than before, and doomed to a life of outlawry and of crime. I was aware that they were each an image of that loveless and hopeless perdition which men once imagined that God had prepared for the souls of the damned, but I could not see the barred windows of those hells in the waning light. I could only see the trees along their walks; their dim lawns and gardens, and the castellated forms of the prisons; and the æsthetic sense, which is careful to keep itself pure from pity, was tickled with an agreeable impression of something old and fair. The dusk thickened, and the vast steamboats which ply between the city and the New England ports on Long Island Sound, and daily convey whole populations of passengers between New York and Boston, began to sweep by silently, swiftly, luminous masses on the black water. Their lights aloft at bow and stern, floated with them like lambent planets; the lights of lesser craft dipped by, and came and went in the distance; the lamps of the nearer and farther shores twinkled into sight, and a peace that ignored all the misery of it, fell upon the scene.

HENRY JAMES

Henry James, whom his friend Howells spoke of as the greatest novelist who ever lived, was born in 1843, the younger brother, by a year, of the celebrated philosopher William James. His father, after whom he was named, was a Swedenborgian thinker who was interesting enough to be mentioned by Morris Raphael Cohen in a chapter on philosophy in the Cambridge History of American Literature. The family, like that of Proust, was one of independent means which derived from a fortune of several million dollars amassed by Henry's grandfather William, who was described as an "Albany business man." The novelist was born in New York City but travelled widely with his family in Europe as a growing boy and had an irregular education in which "dozens of private schools and tutors succeeded one another in bewildering rapidity in New York, not to speak of later instruction in Bonn, and Geneva, in Paris and London." This experience was in line with his father's theory of education, which regarded it as undesirable that a young man should make any commitment to a choice of profession or way of life too early.

The novelist entered Harvard Law School (his brother William, of course, became one of the luminaries of the Harvard faculty), but his most important experiences in Cambridge appear to have been the personal relationships he formed with literary people like Godkin, who edited the newly founded *Nation*, and with Charles Eliot Norton and his family. He was ineligible to serve in the Civil War because of lameness, but the war was brought home to him by the enlistment of two of his brothers.

Though he was intensely devoted to his craft and produced an enormous body of work, he never became a really popular author. He came closest to it perhaps in an early novella, *Daisy Miller*, a sympathetic study of an American girl in a European setting whose pathetic end is said to have brought tears to the eyes of contemporary readers. He tried to reach a wider public in the 1890's by writing for the theater in a bright, witty manner which sometimes, though not often, recalled that of Oscar Wilde, but the only one of his plays to reach the London stage was not successful and when some friends of his were ill-advised enough, at the end of the performance, to call for the author, he was greeted by catcalls from the balcony.

From this experience he reacted by returning to the novel and story and by taking an ever more independent attitude toward his audience, developing in the process that difficult, involved, and abstract style, which became the butt of parodists like Max Beerbohm, made him the center of an impassioned cult (250 members of which commissioned the painter Sargent to do a portrait of him toward the end of his life), and alienated him more and more from the common reader. In *Expression in America*, Ludwig Lewisohn describes this development as follows: "Henry James, starting out with the simplest and most pellucid of styles, hid himself ever more and more in the folds and swathings and integuments of a hieratic manner and a billowing cloud of words. The perspectives of his structural technique, which served to keep the ultimate actualities of his stories and his immediate reactions to them at a safe distance both from himself and from his readers, grew longer and longer until at last one saw his people and his story but at the end of corridors of phantasmagoric extension." Despite this, Lewisohn's final judgment of James was that he was a "master of form, creator of a body of memorable work . . . [and] probably the most eminent man of letters America has yet to show."

This evaluation and the steady, unassailable, literary self-confidence of James himself (which caused him to prophesy that a day would come when his buried works would "kick off their tombstones" all at once) have been increasingly sustained by the verdict of posterity, and the esoteric works of the unpopular author who was "caviare to the general" of the public in his own time have been turned into successful plays and even movies in our time. Forty years ago, Van Wyck Brooks could still write apologetically in the *Encyclopaedia Britannica:* "James's originality, his distinction of style and his fineness of feeling are acknowledged by all and place him very close to the first rank of modern writers." Now he appears to those in literary circles to be even better than that, and Charles R. Anderson, in *American Literary Masters,* is only expressing a consensus from which there are few dissenters when he writes of James that "he produced a body of novels and tales that fill thirty-six volumes yet maintain a remarkably high level of performance. Fully two thirds of this large shelf can be reckoned as first-rate, and half of these rank with the best fictions in English." A century and a quarter after his birth and more than half a century after his death, the world in general seems to be coming round if not precisely to the degree of enthusiasm expressed by Howells yet to something pretty close to it.

The American Scene, from which our selection on the lower East Side is taken, was published in 1907. It is the account of a trip to America, the first in twenty years, that James had taken from England in 1904 at the age of sixty. He was by that time well settled in England where he was to become an English citizen during the First World War in protest against his native country's slowness in coming to the rescue of European civilization. In 1916, England officially recognized his distinction by awarding him the Order of Merit, a few months before his death. These later developments only brought to a head the uneasy relationship which had existed from the beginning between the instinctive aristocratic refinement of James's temperament and the atmosphere of the vulgar democracy in which he had been born.

The estrangement is adequately symbolized by the contemptuous review he wrote for the *Nation* in 1865, fresh out of Harvard, of Whitman's newly published *Drum-Taps:* "Mr. Whitman prides himself especially on the substance—the life—of his poetry. It may be rough, it may be grim, it may be clumsy—such we take to be the author's argument—but it is sincere, it is sublime, it appeals to the soul of man, it is the voice of a people. He tells us . . .

that the words of his book are nothing. To our perception they are everything, and very little at that. . . . It is not enough to be grim and rough and careless; common sense is also necessary, for it is by common sense that we are judged. There exists in even the commonest minds, in literary matters, a certain precise instinct of conservatism, which is very shrewd in detecting wanton eccentricities."

It is only fair to James to note that he lived long enough to be ashamed of this judgment and to try to bury it from public view. He made amends, according to Edith Wharton's autobiography, *A Backward Glance*, by reading aloud from Whitman's work in the company of his friends and he wrote very much more sympathetically of Whitman in his review of the poet's letters to Pete Doyle in *Calamus* when that book appeared in 1898. But his initial misunderstanding of the greatest celebrator of American democracy is not an insignificant or isolated event. Hostility to the unwashed proliferating masses of the immigrants and fear of their potentiality for encouraging the already objectionable money-madness of America and destroying in the process all that he recognized as the finer flowers of its cultural life seem to be the dominant motives of *The American Scene*. If the alien East European Jews alarm him especially, it is because they are just like other Americans, *only more so*. James's most painstaking and massively assiduous biographer, Leon Edel, who is himself Jewish, may derive what comfort he can from James's observation that "the individual Jew [is] more of a concentrated person, savingly possessed of everything that is in him, than any other human, noted at random," but he cannot gloss over the fact that the context of this remark is one of unmitigated trepidation at what the multiplication of the Jews portends for the future of America itself and of the English language and literature. The refuge of the impressionist observer, impatient of more precise and prosaic analysis, is found (as is usually the case) in apocalyptic visions. One of these is horrendous enough to take on a sinister meaning altogether different from the one James intended at the beginning of the century. When he writes of the possible fate awaiting the little people of America who are thriving so prosperously at the present time: "Put it, at the worst, that the

Ogres were to devour them, they were but the more certainly to fatten into food for the Ogres," he inspires the post-holocaust, post-Hiroshima reader with thoughts of which he could hardly have conceived.

Perhaps the cause of James's deficiency as a social analyst lay in his very strength as an analyst of individual psychology, which he summed up in his well-known bit of advice to the writer in *The Art of Fiction:* "Try to be one of the people on whom nothing is lost." But a person upon whom nothing is lost, it may be said, is perhaps also a person upon whom many things great and important might be lost. He might have an extraordinary addiction to trifles, be disoriented and confused and totally lack a sense of direction in the larger issues of life. The difference is that which exists between quantum mechanics and field theory in physics; the very smallest matters in the universe do not appear to be ruled by the same laws as the largest. That may be an offense to logic, but it appears to be so. When it came to the shapes of things to come in our democratic experiment, Whitman took the eagle's-eye view, James the mole's; no wonder the two could hardly understand each other's language, as is indicated not only by James's immediate response to Whitman but by Whitman's succinct characterization of the effect produced on him by James's circumlocutions: "Feathers!" What Whitman might have meant by this descriptive word is illustrated by a typical sentence from *The American Scene:* "During the great loops thrown out by the lasso of observation from the wonder-working motor-car that defied the shrinkage of autumn days, this remained constantly the best formula of the impression and even of the emotion; it sat in the vehicle with us, but spreading its wings to the magnificence of movement, and gathering under them indeed most of the meanings of the picture." Even if you read this over carefully and even if you are informed that the word "this" refers to a phrase in the sentences before and after "the heart of New England," I think it would still be safe to defy you to explain exactly what he means.

But there is no mistaking the feeling which breathes out of his pages about what he calls "the monstrous form of Democracy" or the irony with which he speaks of (the quotation marks are his own) "the working of democratic institutions." James's attitude toward the Jews (anticipated to some extent by Brooks and Henry Adams) marks a kind of watershed in American literary history. It has, of course, nothing to do with the motive of a Cotton Mather to save the souls of those unenlightened by the Christian revelation, it has even less to do with the motivations of men of the eighteenth-century Age of Reason who made the American Revolution or with the prevailing humanitarian attitudes of the century following. It looks forward to the feelings which gained strength in the wake of World War I and the Russian Revolution, with its universal pretensions and threat to all established and traditional institutions, and which found cruder expressions in the correspondence of Theodore Dreiser (unpublished till long after his death) and such a malignant caricature as that of the gangster Meyer Wolfshiem in *The Great Gatsby,* whom Edith Wharton described in a letter to Fitzgerald as the "perfect Jew."

The American Scene

New York really, I think, is all formidable foreground; or, if it be not, there is more than enough of this pressure of the present and the immediate to cut out the close sketcher's work for him. These things are a thick growth all round him, and when I recall the intensity of the material picture in the dense Yiddish quarter, for instance, I wonder at its not having forestalled, on my page, mere musings and, as they will doubtless be called, moonings. There abides with me, ineffaceably, the memory of a summer evening spent there by invitation of a high public functionary domiciled on the spot—to the extreme enhancement of the romantic interest his visitor found him foredoomed to inspire—who was to prove one of the most liberal of hosts and most luminous of guides. I can scarce help it if this brilliant personality, on that occasion the very medium itself through which the whole spectacle showed, so colours my impressions that if I speak, by intention, of the facts that played into them I may really but reflect the rich talk and the general privilege of the hour. That accident moreover must take its place simply as the highest value and the strongest note in the total show—so much did it testify to the quality of appealing, surrounding life. The sense of this quality was already strong in my drive, with a companion, through the long, warm June twilight, from a comparatively conventional neighbourhood; it was the sense, after all, of a great swarming, a swarming that had begun to thicken, infinitely, as soon as we had crossed to the East Side and long before we had got to Rutgers Street. There is no swarm-

Selection from *The American Scene* by Henry James, published by Harper's, New York, 1907.

ing like that of Israel when once Israel has got a start, and the scene here bristled, at every step, with the signs and sounds, immitigable, unmistakable, of a Jewry that had burst all bounds. That it has burst all bounds in New York, almost any combination of figures or of objects taken at hazard sufficiently proclaims; but I remember how the rising waters, on this summer night, rose, to the imagination, even above the housetops and seemed to sound their murmur to the pale distant stars. It was as if we had been thus, in the crowded, hustled roadway, where multiplication, multiplication of everything, was the dominant note, at the bottom of some vast sallow aquarium in which innumerable fish, of overdeveloped proboscis, were to bump together, forever, amid heaped spoils of the sea.

The children swarmed above all—here was multiplication with a vengeance; and the number of very old persons, of either sex, was almost equally remarkable; the very old persons being in equal vague occupation of the doorstep, pavement, curbstone, gutter, roadway, and every one alike using the street for overflow. As overflow, in the whole quarter, is the main fact of life—I was to learn later on that, with the exception of some shy corner of Asia, no district in the world known to the statistician has so many inhabitants to the yard—the scene hummed with the human presence beyond any I had ever faced in quest even of refreshment; producing part of the impression, moreover, no doubt, as a direct consequence of the intensity of the Jewish aspect. This, I think, makes the individual Jew more of a concentrated person, savingly possessed of everything that is in him, than any other human, noted at random—or is it simply, rather, that the unsurpassed strength of the race permits of the chopping into myriads of fine fragments without loss of race-quality? There are small strange animals, known to natural history, snakes or worms, I believe, who, when cut into pieces, wriggle away contentedly and live in the snippet as completely as in the whole. So the denizens of the New York Ghetto, heaped as thick as the splinters on the table of a glass-blower, had each, like the fine glass particle, his or her individual share of the whole hard glitter of Israel. This diffused intensity, as I have called it, causes any array of Jews to resemble (if I may be allowed another image) some long nocturnal street where every window in every house shows a maintained light. The advanced age of so many of the figures, the ubiquity of the children, carried out in fact this analogy; they were all there for race, and not, as it were, for reason: that excess of lurid meaning, in some of the old men's and old women's faces in particular, would have been absurd, in the conditions, as a really directed attention—it could only be the gathered past of Israel mechanically pushing through. The way, at the same time, this chapter of history did, all that evening, seem to push, was a matter that made the "ethnic" apparition again sit like a skeleton at the feast. It was fairly as if I could see the spectre grin while the talk of the hour gave me, across the board, facts and figures, chapter and verse, for the extent of the Hebrew conquest of New York. With a reverence for intellect, one should doubtless have drunk in tribute to an intellectual people; but I remember being at no time more conscious of that merely portentous element, in the aspects of American growth, which reduces to inanity any marked dismay quite as much as any high elation. The portent is one of too many—you always come back, as I have hinted, with your easier gasp, to *that:* it will be time enough to sigh or to shout when the relation of the particular appearance to all the other relations shall have cleared itself up. Phantasmagoric for me, accordingly, in a high degree, are the interesting hours I here glance at content to remain—setting in this respect, I recognize, an excellent example to all the rest of the New York phantasmagoria. Let me speak of the remainder only as phantasmagoric too, so that I may both the more kindly recall it and the sooner have done with it.

I have not done, however, with the impression of that large evening in the Ghetto; there was too much in the vision, and it has left too much the sense of a rare experience. For what did it all really come to but that one had seen with one's eyes the New Jerusalem on earth? What less than that could it all have been, in its far-spreading light and its celestial serenity of multiplication? There it was, there it is, and when I think of the dark, foul, stifling Ghettos of other remembered cities, I shall think by the same stroke of the city of redemption, and evoke in particular the rich Rutgers Street perspective—rich, so peculiarly, for the eye, in

73

that complexity of fire-escapes with which each house-front bristles and which gives the whole vista so modernized and appointed
a look. Omnipresent in the "poor" regions, this neat applied
machinery has, for the stranger, a common side with the electric
light and the telephone, suggests the distance achieved from the
old Jerusalem. (These frontal iron ladders and platforms, by the
way, so numerous throughout New York, strike more New York
notes than can be parenthetically named—and among them perhaps most sharply the note of the ease with which, in the terrible
town, on opportunity, "architecture" goes by the board; but the
appearance to which they often most conduce is that of the spa-
ciously organized cage for the nimbler class of animals in some
great zoological garden. This general analogy is irresistible—it
seems to offer, in each district, a little world of bars and perches
and swings for human squirrels and monkeys. The very name of
architecture perishes, for the fire-escapes look like abashed
afterthoughts, staircases and communications forgotten in the construction; but the inhabitants lead, like the squirrels and monkeys, all the merrier life.) It was while I hung over the prospect
from the windows of my friend, however, the presiding genius of
the district, and it was while, at a later hour, I proceeded in his
company, and in that of a trio of contributive fellow-pilgrims,
from one "characteristic" place of public entertainment to another: it was during this rich climax, I say, that the city of
redemption was least to be taken for anything less than it was. The
windows, while we sat at meat, looked out on a swarming little
square in which an ant-like population darted to and fro; the
square consisted in part of a "district" public garden, or public
lounge rather, one of those small backwaters or refuges, artfully
economized for rest, here and there, in the very heart of the New
York whirlpool, and which spoke louder than anything else of a
Jerusalem disinfected. What spoke loudest, no doubt, was the
great overtowering School which formed a main boundary and in
the shadow of which we all comparatively crouched.

But the School must not lead me on just yet—so colossally has
its presence still to loom for us; that presence which profits so,
for predominance, in America, by the failure of concurrent and
competitive presences, the failure of any others looming at all on

the same scale save that of Business, those in particular of a visible Church, a visible State, a visible Society, a visible Past; those of the many visibilities, in short, that warmly cumber the ground in older countries. Yet it also spoke loud that my friend was quartered, for the interest of the thing (from his so interesting point of view), in a "tenement-house"; the New Jerusalem would so have triumphed, had it triumphed nowhere else, in the fact that this charming little structure *could* be ranged, on the wonderful little square, under that invidious head. On my asking to what latent vice it owed its stigma, I was asked in return if it didn't sufficiently pay for its name by harbouring some five-and-twenty families. But this, exactly, was the way it testified—this circumstance of the simultaneous enjoyment by five-and-twenty families, on "tenement" lines, of conditions so little sordid, so highly "evolved." I remember the evolved fire-proof staircase, a thing of scientific surfaces, impenetrable to the microbe, and above all plated, against side friction, with white marble of a goodly grain. The white marble was surely the New Jerusalem note, and we followed that note, up and down the district, the rest of the evening, through more happy changes than I may take time to count. What struck me in the flaring streets (over and beyond the everywhere insistent, defiant, unhumorous, exotic face) was the blaze of the shops addressed to the New Jerusalem wants and the splendour with which these were taken for granted; the only thing indeed a little ambiguous was just this look of the trap too brilliantly, too candidly baited for the wary side of Israel itself. It is not *for* Israel, in general, that Israel so artfully shines—yet its being moved to do so, at last, in that luxurious style, might be precisely the grand side of the city of redemption. Who can ever tell, moreover, in any conditions and in presence of any apparent anomaly, what the genius of Israel may, or may not, really be "up to"?

The grateful way to take it all, at any rate, was with the sense of its coming back again to the inveterate rise, in the American air, of every value, and especially of the lower ones, those most subject to multiplication; such a wealth of meaning did this keep appearing to pour into the value and function of the country at large. Importances are all strikingly shifted and reconstituted, in the

United States, for the visitor attuned, from far back, to "European" importances; but I think of no other moment of my total impression as so sharply working over my own benighted vision of them. The scale, in this light of the New Jerusalem, seemed completely rearranged; or, to put it more simply, the wants, the gratifications, the aspirations of the "poor," as expressed in the shops (which were the shops of the "poor"), denoted a new style of poverty; and this new style of poverty, from street to street, stuck out of the possible purchasers, one's jostling fellow-pedestrians, and made them, to every man and woman, individual throbs in the larger harmony. One can speak only of what one has seen, and there were grosser elements of the sordid and the squalid that I doubtless never saw. That, with a good deal of observation and of curiosity, I should have failed of this, the country over, affected me as by itself something of an indication. To miss that part of the spectacle, or to know it only by its having so unfamiliar a pitch, was an indication that made up for a great many others. It is when this one in particular is forced home to you—this immense, vivid *general* lift of poverty and general appreciation of the living unit's paying property in himself—that the picture seems most to clear and the way to jubilation most to open. For it meets you there, at every turn, as the result most definitely attested. You are as constantly reminded, no doubt, that these rises in enjoyed value shrink and dwindle under the icy breath of Trusts and the weight of the new remorseless monopolies that operate as no madnesses of ancient personal power thrilling us on the historic page ever operated; the living unit's property in himself becoming more and more merely such a property as may consist with a relation to properties overwhelmingly greater and that allow the asking of no questions and the making, for co-existence with them, of no conditions. But that, in the fortunate phrase, is another story, and will be altogether, evidently, a new and different drama. There is such a thing, in the United States, it is hence to be inferred, as freedom to grow up to be blighted, and it may be the only freedom in store for the smaller fry of future generations. If it is accordingly of the smaller fry I speak, and of how large they massed on that evening of endless admonitions, this will be because I caught them thus in their comparative humility and at an early stage of their American growth. The life-thread has, I suppose, to be of a certain thickness for the great shears of Fate to feel for it. Put it, at the worst, that the Ogres were to devour them, they were but the more certainly to fatten into food for the Ogres.

Their dream, at all events, as I noted it, was meanwhile sweet and undisguised—nowhere sweeter than in the half-dozen picked beer-houses and cafés in which our ingenuous *enquête,* that of my fellow-pilgrims and I, wound up. These establishments had each been selected for its playing off some facet of the jewel, and they wondrously testified, by their range and their individual colour, to the spread of that lustre. It was a pious rosary of which I should like to tell each bead, but I must let the general sense of the adventure serve. Our successive stations were in no case of the "seamy" order, an inquiry into seaminess having been unanimously pronounced futile, but each had its separate social connotation, and it was for the number and variety of these connotations, and their individual plenitude and prosperity, to set one thinking. Truly the Yiddish world was a vast world, with its own deeps and complexities, and what struck one above all was that it sat there at its cups (and in no instance vulgarly the worse for them) with a sublimity of good conscience that took away the breath, a protrusion of elbow never aggressive, but absolutely proof against jostling. It was the incurable man of letters under the skin of one of the party who gasped, I confess; for it was in the light of letters, that is in the light of our language as literature has hitherto known it, that one stared at this all-unconscious impudence of the agency of future ravage. The man of letters, in the United States, has his own difficulties to face and his own current to stem—for dealing with which his liveliest inspiration may be, I think, that they are still very much his own, even in an Americanized world, and that more than elsewhere they press him to intimate communion with his honour. For that honour, the honour that sits astride of the consecrated English tradition, to his mind, quite as old knighthood astride of its caparisoned charger, the dragon most rousing, over the land, the proper spirit of St. George, is just this immensity of the alien presence climbing higher and higher, climbing itself into the very light of publicity.

I scarce know why, but I saw it that evening as in some dim

dawn of that promise to its own consciousness, and perhaps this was precisely what made it a little exasperating. Under the impression of the mere mob the question doesn't come up, but in these haunts of comparative civility we saw the mob sifted and strained, and the exasperation was the sharper, no doubt, because what the process had left most visible was just the various possibilities of the waiting spring of intelligence. Such elements constituted the germ of a "public," and it was impossible (possessed of a sensibility worth speaking of) to be exposed to them without feeling how new a thing under the sun the resulting public would be. That was where one's "lettered" anguish came in—in the turn of one's eye from face to face for some betrayal of a prehensile hook for the linguistic tradition as one had known it. Each warm, lighted and supplied circle, each group of served tables and smoked pipes and fostered decencies and unprecedented accents, beneath the extravagant lamps, took on thus, for the brooding critic, a likeness to that terrible modernized and civilized room in the Tower of London, haunted by the shade of Guy Fawkes, which had more than once formed part of the scene of the critic's taking tea there. In this chamber of the present urbanities the wretched man had been stretched on the rack, and the critic's ear (how else should it have been a critic's?) could still always catch, in pauses of talk, the faint groan of his ghost. Just so the East Side cafés—and increasingly as their place in the scale was higher—showed to my inner sense, beneath their bedizenment, as torture-rooms of the living idiom; the piteous gasp of which at the portent of lacerations to come could reach me in any drop of the surrounding Accent of the Future. The accent of the very ultimate future, in the States, may be destined to become the most beautiful on the globe and the very music of humanity (here the "ethnic" synthesis shrouds itself thicker than ever); but whatever we shall know it for, certainly, we shall not know it for English—in any sense for which there is an existing literary measure.

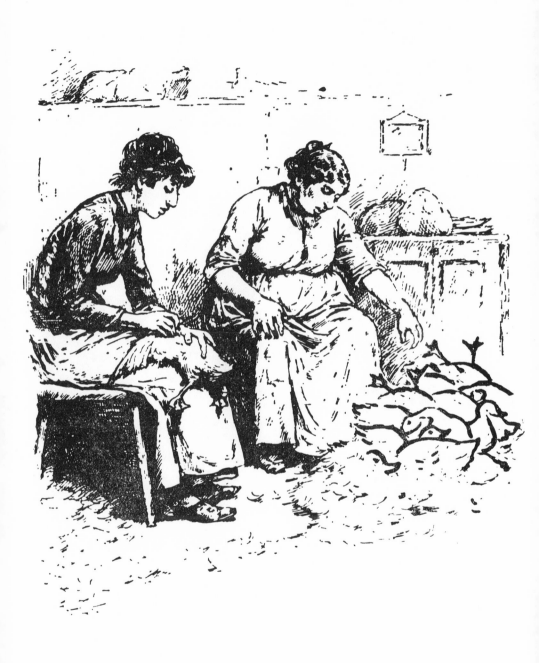

LINCOLN STEFFENS

Joseph Lincoln Steffens, the
American political writer and journalist, was born in San Francisco on April 6, 1866, the son of Joseph and Elizabeth Louisa
(Symes) Steffens. He spent his boyhood on a ranch near Sacra-
mento, where he learned to be a good horseman and also indulged
a taste for drawing. He was sent to a military school from which
he was expelled for "drunkenness." His father then secured as
tutor for him an Oxford man who coached him for the University
of California and really initiated him into an intellectual life.
Steffens got his Ph.B. degree from the university in 1889 and
then went to Europe, where he studied for three years at Berlin,
Heidelberg, Leipzig, and the Sorbonne.

He came back with a wife, Josephine Boutecou, whom he had
married in London in 1891. He got a job as police reporter for the
New York Evening Post, of which he later became city editor. At
this time he met Theodore Roosevelt and Jacob Riis and became
interested in social questions. From 1898 to 1902, he was city editor of the reorganized *Commercial Advertiser* and from there
went to *McClure's Magazine,* of which he was managing editor
for four years. He became very well known among the so-called
"muckrakers," who included Ida Tarbell, Finley Peter Dunne
(Mr. Dooley) and Ray Stannard Baker. A series of sensational
political exposés were gathered together into an even more sensational book, which Steffens entitled *The Shame of the Cities.* He
made an attempt, with the help of Edward A. Filene, to clean up
the corruption of the city government of Boston, but nothing
finally came of it.

In 1919, he served on the secret Bullitt mission to Soviet Russia, a visit that was to have a great effect upon his general political outlook. In a famous phrase, which was much quoted by the numerous fellow travellers of Communism in the thirties, he declared that in Russia he had seen the future, and it "works." In the final years of his life (he died on August 9, 1936) he became affiliated with the Communist party of the United States. His manner as a reporter impressed John Chamberlain and Albert Jay Nock, who both described him, according to *Twentieth Century Authors,* as a kind of "Socrates of the sanctum," who delighted in questioning everybody and everything with an apparent naïveté but actually with much shrewdness. One of the secrets of the charm he exerted even upon some of those whom he most opposed was that he liked people, including what he called "honest crooks" and "good bad capitalists." He said: "Intelligence is what I'm aiming at, not honesty!"

Autobiography

Dew is a shower of jewels—
in the country, and as it melts in the morning sun it sweetens the
air. Not in a city. Police headquarters was in a tenement neighborhood, which seemed to steam on warm nights and sweat by day. I
can remember still the damp, smelly chill of the asphalt pavement
that greeted me when I came to my office in the early mornings.
The tenements stank, the alleys puffed forth the stenches of the
night. Slatternly women hung out of the windows to breathe and
to gossip or quarrel across the courts; idle men and boys hung,
half dressed, over the old iron fences or sat recovering from the
night on the stoops of the houses which once had been the fine
homes of the old families long since moved uptown. There was a
business man in a new building next door to headquarters. He
was a handsome, well-dressed wholesale dealer in brass fixtures
and plumbers' supplies, and he may have thought he was waiting
for buyers, but he was looking for something to happen, like the
other neighbors. When a Black Maria drove up and discharged a
load of thieves, prostitutes, broken strikers, or gambling-
implements, he joined the crowd of loafers, men, women, and
children, who gathered to enjoy the sight.

I looked for him, I looked for all the bums, when I turned into
Mulberry Street; they were signs of expectancy from which I
could guess whether there was news to write. If they were idle I
might have time to breathe. I could not be sure, however, till I
saw and spoke to the patrolman who acted as doorman of police
headquarters. He was always on the stoop, idle, humorous, and

Selection from Lincoln Steffens' *Autobiography*, published by Harcourt
Brace, New York, 1931.

Irish. He could not be surprised; he was always expectant and aware. I had to ask him, "Anything doing, Pat?"

"Not yet," he would say, and nodding his wise old head up and down the street at the reporters, bums, business man, and women at their doors and windows, "They're all out, you see."

If these were not on post, if the reporters were in their offices and the neighbors stood in groups, Pat would answer my question with "Well, as you see, they're all telling—something." And slowly, with proper dignity and police mystery, he would tell me enough to judge whether it was a story I had to write. If I was in doubt, Riis's boy, Max, would settle it.

"What's up, Max?"

"Oh, nothing for you. A slum murder." Or "a roof chase after a thief," or "a baby fell off a fire-escape," or "a gang of toughs broke fences, door-bells, windows all along East Thirty-fifth Street."

The last was a common event. It was as unimportant as similar student pranks are in a college town. Reporters wrote it up only when they had nothing else to report and had to send in something to justify a day of poker. I wrote it once—twice. I had begun to break through my instructions to stick to police politics and Parkhurst exposures and ignore criminal news. I wrote crimes now and then, and the eagerness with which my city editor received them and the cautious way he slipped them into obscure parts of the paper encouraged me to believe that he wanted me gradually to get and so report regular police news that he could broaden the narrow scope of *Evening Post* news. He had been himself a police reporter; he knew the many kinds of stories that came out at headquarters, and he thought that Mr. Godkin would not mind if it was "written right"—not sensationally. Also he knew that I could not help trying it—somehow.

I took from Max that day the exact, outrageous details of the destructive raid of a gang of toughs in East Thirty-fifth Street and I described cheerfully, almost joyously, the breakages those drunks wreaked; I wrote it as nearly as I could in the jolly spirit of the night out. Max was a born seer; he had it all, and I must have reported it with his inspiration and his smile, for it was printed, and a few days later Wright called me down to the office and said that "the editor" had been receiving a stream of indignant letters asking how a paper like the *Post* could report such an outrage against order and property without a single syllable of indignation. I was so flattered that Wright was puzzled and rather angry. I had to remind him that there were two ways to report an incident like that: to express "our" indignation or to arouse the readers' rage; and that I thought the readers' emotion was more literary and more effective than ours.

"Such outrages happen frequently," I said. "The next time one occurs I will write it as an outrage instead of a descriptive narrative, and you will see that no reader will write to us; they will all be satisfied." And I did that. I began my next story, "An outrageous series of depredations was committed by a gang of drunken young hoodlums—" and all through the narrative I sprinkled denunciation. Not a letter, no protest; Wright was convinced, and he convinced Godkin that the editor did not always know the difference between a report and an editorial and that a description is often more editorial in effect than a Godkin editorial. Best of all, "we" let me report more.

Wright's wish and my ambition was to "do" a murder. One day as I was standing beside the doorman waiting for something to happen, we saw a reporter come running out of the basement and dart across into his office. The doorman winked at me and I stepped down to the telegraph bureau. A woman had been killed in Mulberry Bend. I came out and called, "Max!" Out he ran from his office, and we hurried down to the address in Little Italy. There was a crowd standing watching some children dancing beautifully around an organ-grinder who was playing a waltz.

"There's your story," said Max, pointing at the street scene. "Mine is inside."

Max understood. I went inside with him. We saw the dead woman, the blood, the wretched tenement apartment, and we talked to the neighbors, who told us how the murderer came into the court with the organ-grinder, and while the organ played and the children danced, he had seen the woman's face at the window, recognized her, rushed up, and cut her all to pieces; the crowd gathered and were about to beat the man to death when the police came, saved and arrested him. The poker-playing reporters came tearing up, asked for names, ages, and—details. Theirs was the sensational story of the day, all blood and no dancing. Riis wrote it as a melodrama with a moral, an old cry of his: "Mulberry Bend must go." And, by the way, it went. Such was the power of Riis! There's a small park now where Mulberry Bend was.

I wrote the murder as a descriptive sketch of Italian character, beginning with the dance music, bringing the murder in among the children whose cries called the mob; the excitement, the sudden rage, the saving arrest; and ending with the peaceful after-scene of the children dancing in the street, with the mob smiling and forgetting out in the street.

I saw and heard just such a story in Naples long afterward. Lying abed in the front room of the Hotel Santa Lucia, I was listening to the singers and players entertaining the late diners at the fish restaurants on the quay. One tenor sang high and clear above the rest; a pure, sweet voice, it rose over all the scene and seemed to abash all the other music. The whole dock grew quiet to listen. A victory; and the victor profited by, he seemed to abuse, his power. I could hear, I could feel, him swagger and strut, till a baritone in a boat lifted the same aria, took it away from the tenor, who tried to carry on, but hesitated, halted. The baritone laughed, a musical, a gleeful, provoking laugh. The challenge in it roused the tenor, who sang again, the "Santa Lucia," and we listened; I mean that the whole bay turned to him to hear, and the baritone too. A few thrilling bars and the tenor slipped, a false and overdrawn high note, and the baritone mocked it, laughed, and joining the tenor, sang with him, supporting him to the end. The tenor sang another, and another, the baritone playing him, now in unison, now the second; the two made glorious music, but it was a clinch. The baritone—a fisherman putting his boat in order; I got up, looked out, and saw him—the unprofessional singer corrected, helped, and—he spoiled parts of *Pagliacci* beautifully. His was the purer voice, his the more perfect mastery of the music. He yielded only when he liked, when he had to attend to his nets, to his boat. Sometimes the tenor had it alone for a whole song. I tried, I must have slept. Shouts wakened me, the excited cries and curses of a scuffle. Leaping to the window, I

86

saw a writhing crowd on the wide stone stairway down into the water. It was a fight; I could see blows struck, hands flashing, up and down. The police came. . . . There was silence. The diners moved on, the boatmen went back into their boats, the crowd melted. They had seen a stabbing; an arrest, an ambulance call; they had taken sides, judged, and gone about their own businesses. In the dead quiet outside I went back to bed, but before I could sleep I heard a voice pipe up, a few notes of song, which, after a moment, another voice picked up and finished. By dawn the Bay of Naples was singing again, the dock was passing a bar from one opera, and laughing, matching it with a run from another, which made harmony. At sunrise when I glanced out, the sparkling waters and the villainous Neapolitans were shining as innocently as the sun himself.

The *Post* printed a murder, a mere mean murder, as news, and there was no news in it; only life. "We" published crime after that, all sorts of sensational stuff. Why not? Nobody noticed it, as crime. I soon found out that by going with the reporters to a fire or the scene of an accident was a way to see the town and the life of the town.

A synagogue that burned down during a service introduced me to the service; I attended another synagogue, asked questions, and realized that it was a bit of the Old Testament repeated after thousands of years, unchanged. And so I described that service and other services. They fascinated me, those old practices, and the picturesque customs and laws of the old orthodox Jews from Russia and Poland. Max, an East Side Jew himself, told me about them; I read up and talked to funny old, fine rabbis about them, and about their conflicts with their Americanized children. The *Post* observed all the holy days of the Ghetto. There were advance notices of their coming, with descriptions of the preparations and explanations of their sacred, ancient, biblical meaning, and then an account of them as I saw these days and nights observed in the homes and the churches of the poor. A queer mixture of comedy, tragedy, orthodoxy, and revelation, they interested our Christian readers. The uptown Jews complained now and then. Mr. Godkin himself required me once to call personally upon a socially prominent Jewish lady who had written to the

editor asking why so much space was given to the ridiculous performances of the ignorant, foreign East Side Jews and none to the
uptown Hebrews. I told her. I had the satisfaction of telling her
about the comparative beauty, significance, and character of the
uptown and downtown Jews. I must have talked well, for she
threatened and tried to have me fired, as she put it. Fortunately,
the editorial writers were under pressure also from prominent
Jews to back up their side of a public controversy over the black-
balling of a rich Jew by an uptown social club. "We" were fair to
the Jews, editorially, but personally irritated. I was not "fired"; I
was sent out to interview the proprietor of a hotel which excluded
Jews, and he put his case in a very few words.

"I won't have one," he said. "I have had my experience and so
learned that if you let one in because he is exceptional and fine,
he will bring in others who are not exceptional, etc. By and by
they will occupy the whole house, when the Christians leave. And
then, when the Christians don't come any more, the Jews quit
you to go where the Christians have gone, and there you are with
an empty or a second-class house."

It would have been absurd to discharge me since I at that time
was almost a Jew. I had become as infatuated with the Ghetto as
eastern boys were with the wild west, and nailed a mazuza on my
office door; I went to the synagogue on all the great Jewish holy
days; on Yom Kippur I spent the whole twenty-four hours fasting
and going from one synagogue to another. The music moved me
most, but I knew and could follow with the awful feelings of a
Jew the beautiful old ceremonies of the ancient orthodox services. My friends laughed at me; especially the Jews among them
scoffed. "You are more Jewish than us Jews," they said, and since
I have traveled I realize the absurdity of the American who is
more French than the French, more German than the Kaiser. But
there were some respecters of my respect. When Israel Zangwill,
the author of *Tales of the Ghetto*, came from London to visit New
York, he heard about me from Jews and asked me to be his guide
for a survey of the East Side; and he saw and he went home and
wrote *The Melting Pot.*

The tales of the New York Ghetto were heart-breaking comedies
of the tragic conflict between the old and the new, the very old

and the very new; in many matters, all at once: religion, class, clothes, manners, customs, language, culture. We all know the difference between youth and age, but our experience is between two generations. Among the Russian and other eastern Jewish families in New York it was an abyss of many generations; it was between parents out of the Middle Ages, sometimes out of the Old Testament days hundreds of years B.C., and the children of the streets of New York today. We saw it everywhere all the time. Responding to a reported suicide, we would pass a synagogue where a score or more of boys were sitting hatless in their old clothes, smoking cigarettes on the steps outside, and their fathers, all dressed in black, with their high hats, uncut beards, and temple curls, were going into the synagogues, tearing their hair and rending their garments. The reporters stopped to laugh; and it was comic; the old men, in their thrift, tore the lapels of their coats very carefully, a very little, but they wept tears, real tears. It was a revolution. Their sons were rebels against the law of Moses; they were lost souls, lost to God, the family, and to Israel of old. The police did not understand or sympathize. If there was a fight— and sometimes the fathers did lay hands on their sons, and the tough boys did biff their fathers in the eye; which brought out all the horrified elders of the whole neighborhood and all the sullen youth—when there was a "riot call," the police would rush in and club now the boys, now the parents, and now, in their Irish exasperation, both sides, bloodily and in vain. I used to feel that the blood did not hurt, but the tears did, the weeping and gnashing of teeth of the old Jews who were doomed and knew it. Two, three, thousand years of continuous devotion, courage, and suffering for a cause lost in a generation.

"Oh, Meester Report!" an old woman wailed one evening. "Come into my house and see my childer, my little girls." She seized and pulled me in (me and, I think, Max) up the stairs, weeping, into her clean, dark room, one room, where her three little girls were huddled at the one rear window, from which they— and we—could see a prostitute serving a customer. "*Da, se'en Sie,* there they are watching, always they watch." As the children rose at sight of us and ran away, the old woman told us how her children had always to see that beastly sight. "They count the men who come of a night," she said. "Ninety-three one night." (I shall never forget that number.) "My oldest girl says she will go into that business when she grows up; she says it's a good business, easy, and you can dress and eat and live."

"Why don't you pull down your curtain?" I asked.

"We have no curtain," she wept. "I hang up my dress across, but the childer when I sleep or go out, they crowd under it to see."

"Ask the woman to pull her blind."

"I have," she shrieked. "Oh, I have begged her on my knees, and she won't."

I went over and asked the girl to draw her curtain.

"I won't," she cried in a sudden rage. "That old woman had me raided, and the police—you know it—you know how they hound us now for Parkhurst. They drove me from where I was and I hid in here. That old woman, she sent for the police, and now I have to pay—big—to stay here."

"All right, all right," I shouted to down her mad shrieks of rage. "But her children look—"

"I don't care," the girl yelled back. "It serves her right, that old devil. I will get even. I will ruin her nasty children, as she says."

I threatened to "make" the police close her up, and down she came, all in tears.

"Don't, please don't, Mr. Reporter," she cried. "They'll run me out, the cops will, for you; I know; and I'll have a hell of a time to get found again by my customers. I'm doing well here now again; I can soon open a house maybe and get some girls and be respectable myself if—"

So we compromised. She pinned up a blanket on her window, and I promised not to have her driven out. When I came out into the street there was a patrolman at the door.

"What's the kick?" he asked.

I told him briefly all about it; he knew, nodded. "What's to be done?" he asked.

"Nothing," I answered hastily. "I have fixed it. Don't do anything. It's all right now."

It wasn't, of course. Nothing was all right. Neither in this case, nor in prostitution generally, nor in the strikes—is there any right —or wrong; not that the police could do, nor I, nor the *Post*, nor Dr. Parkhurst. It was, it is, all a struggle between conflicting interests, between two blind opposite sides, neither of which is right or wrong.

JACOB RIIS

Jacob Riis, editor, author, journalist, reformer, and photographer extraordinary of lower East Side life, was born in Ribe, Denmark, in 1849, the son of a teacher in the Ribe Latin School, which Riis attended from 1858 to 1864. He lived to become the man whom his friend Theodore Roosevelt (for whose election as Governor of New York State he had worked hard) called "the most useful citizen of New York" and "the ideal American."

As a child he knew Hans Christian Andersen. His father (reversing the tradition by which parents oppose the choice of their children for artistic careers and wish them to be more practical) wanted him to embark on a literary career, but Jacob decided to take up carpentry instead. Evidently he found few opportunities to satisfy him in his native land in either the higher vocation or the lower one, for at the age of twenty-one, in the year 1870, he sailed for the United States.

He landed in New York during a time of widespread unemployment, and finding no work there travelled to Pittsburgh, where he built huts for miners and for a while tried his hand at mining himself. In July 1870, after he had once again taken up his old trade of carpentry, word came that France had declared war on Prussia and that Denmark was expected to join forces with France. Riis then returned to New York and notified the Danish Consul that in the event of war he wished to be returned to Denmark to fight. He then wandered pennilessly around New York for quite a while, on one occasion spurning a dollar handout from

Charles A. Dana, who was to become his employer years later, because the latter had made a slighting remark while offering the money to him: "Go get your breakfast, and better give up the war!"

He worked at a brickyard for six weeks, then got a job on a French steamer, which, however, unfortunately sailed away before he could come aboard. His next adventure was joining a band of tramps that was travelling South. He got as far as Philadelphia, where he found a shelter of sorts with the Danish Consul and then wandered back to New York State. In Buffalo, he finally decided he would adopt an "intellectual" profession and become a reporter, but the *Buffalo Courier and Express* turned him down. He then went to Jamestown, New York, where he got a job selling furniture and was quite successful at it. At this time (1873 —Riis rarely gives precise dates in his memoirs), he received a letter that his Danish sweetheart, Elizabeth, was to be married to someone else.

In replying to a newspaper notice, he got a job as city editor of a Long Island City weekly, the *Review*, but when he found he could not collect his wages he quit. For a second time he wandered around New York penniless and literally starving when, by pure luck, he met an old acquaintance who got him a job at a news agency—the New York News Association at 23 Park Row. On May 20, 1874, he landed a job with the *South Brooklyn News*, a paper founded by South Brooklyn politicians to further their interests. Two weeks later he was named editor, but the paper soon went bankrupt. Riis managed to buy the paper for $1,650 —in promissory notes, not in cash—and became its editor, reporter, publisher, and advertising agent.

He then reports falling under the influence of a fire-and-brimstone Methodist preacher, Brother Simmons, and under this religious influence surprising the town by advocating civic reform in his newspaper. This happened, in his own words, "in the days of Grant's second term, and the disgrace of it was foul." Pretty soon, he decided to sell his paper, got back five times the purchase price he had invested and promptly sailed for Denmark to marry Elizabeth, who had somehow managed to hold out and wait for him.

Riis returned to America and invested his money in a stereopticon (slide lantern) business and travelled about the country using it for advertising purposes. Eventually he returned to New York and got a job with the *Tribune* as a reporter. This was in 1878, and he calls his job of police reporter on this paper "the beginning of my career." Later on, he transferred to the *New York Evening Sun*. His first efforts as a civic reformer occurred around this time. He felt driven to investigate the New York Police Department because of a feeling of outrage against a police sergeant who had killed a mongrel dog that had befriended Riis years before when he was destitute. This investigation resulted in his initiating a campaign to eliminate so-called police lodging rooms, which were used at the time to house the poor and which Riis found to be in the most wretched condition. This campaign was destined for eventual success when he persuaded his friend Theodore Roosevelt as Police Commissioner to shut them down in 1895.

In the year 1879, he began to concern himself with the tenement-house question. In 1884, he copyrighted the title of his famous book *How the Other Half Lives,* though the book itself was not to be written for another two years. Riis in his memoir, *The Making of an American,* tells of the beginning of his career as a photographer: "It was upon my midnight trips with the Sanitary Police that the wish kept cropping up in me that there were some way of putting before the people what I saw there." In this period he also became interested in the wretched conditions prevailing in the Mulberry Bend—a row of flophouses—and was instrumental in having it converted into a park.

Though he was assiduously taking photographs now, he was unsuccessful for quite a time in selling them to the magazines. One of the editors of *Scribner's,* however, was interested enough in a Riis photograph to talk to him about it. "As a result of that talk I wrote an article that appeared in the Christmas *Scribner's,* 1889, under the title 'How the Other Half Lives' and . . . made an instant impression on the public." On page 308 of his autobiography, he reproduces a facsimile of a letter written to him by James Russell Lowell on November 21, 1890, in response to this article and the book of the same title, which was printed shortly afterward and became quite popular, as did also his second book, *Children of the Poor.*

Riis was appointed by Mayor Strong of New York City as Secretary of the Small Parks Committee. He wrote an article for *Century Magazine*, "The Making of Thieves in New York," which dealt with the despicable way in which New York officials handled juvenile offenders. When the Spanish-American War broke out in 1898, he wanted to join Teddy Roosevelt's Rough Riders but did not find it possible to do so. Of his friendship with Roosevelt, he writes: "as for Roosevelt, few were nearer to him I fancy, than I, even at Albany." It was not an idle or vain boast. His memoir concludes with the account of another return to Denmark to visit his aging mother and a reminiscence of the years he spent with his wife.

Among his many useful accomplishments, he started in 1888 the Jacob A. Riis Neighborhood House for social work. He wrote in his book *The Battle with the Slum* with justifiable pride: "New York is a many times cleaner and better city today than it was twenty or even ten years ago. Then I was able to grasp easily the whole plan for wresting it from the neglect and indifference that had put us where we were. It was chiefly, almost wholly, remedial in its scope. Now it is preventive, and no ten men could gather all the threads and hold them. We have made, are making, headway, and no Tammany has the power to stop us." His later years were spent largely in writing, lecturing and social work. He died in 1914 on his farm in Barre, Maine. His memory is honored in New York by a settlement house, a state park and bathing beach in the Rockaways, and a housing project. Perhaps it may be worth mentioning as a curiosity that Gertrude Stein seems to have taken the title of her second book, *The Making of Americans* (which followed her well-known book *Three Lives*), from the imaginative title which Riis gave to his own memoirs.

How the Other Half Lives

Lhe tenements grow taller, and the gaps in their ranks close up rapidly as we cross the Bowery and, leaving Chinatown and the Italians behind, invade the Hebrew quarter. Baxter Street, with its interminable rows of old clothes shops and its brigades of pullers-in—nicknamed "the Bay" in honor, perhaps, of the tars who lay to there after a cruise to stock up their togs, or maybe after the "schooners" of beer plentifully bespoke in that latitude—Bayard Street, with its synagogues and its crowds, gave us a foretaste of it. No need of asking here where we are. The jargon of the street, the signs of the sidewalk, the manner and dress of the people, their unmistakable physiognomy, betray their race at every step. Men with queer skullcaps, venerable beard, and the outlandish long-skirted kaftan of the Russian Jew, elbow the ugliest and the handsomest women in the land. The contrast is startling. The old women are hags; the young, houris. Wives and mothers at sixteen, at thirty they are old. So thoroughly has the chosen people crowded out the Gentiles in the Tenth Ward that, when the great Jewish holidays come around every year, the public schools in the district have practically to close up. Of their thousands of pupils scarce a handful come to school. Nor is there any suspicion that the rest are playing hookey. They stay honestly home to celebrate. There is no mistaking it: we are in Jewtown.

It is said that nowhere in the world are so many people crowded together on a square mile as here. The average five-story tenement adds a story or two to its stature in Ludlow Street and

Chapter from *How the Other Half Lives* by Jacob Riis, published by Scribner's, New York, 1902.

an extra building on the rear lot, and yet the sign "To Let" is the rarest of all there. Here is one seven stories high. The sanitary policeman whose beat this is will tell you that it contains thirty-six families, but the term has a widely different meaning here and on the avenues. In this house, where a case of small-pox was reported, there were fifty-eight babies and thirty-eight children that were over five years of age. In Essex Street two small rooms in a six-story tenement were made to hold a "family" of father and mother, twelve children and six boarders. The boarder plays as important a part in the domestic economy of Jewtown as the lodger in the Mulberry Street Bend. These are samples of the packing of the population that has run up the record here to the rate of three hundred and thirty thousand per square mile. The densest crowding of Old London, I pointed out before, never got beyond a hundred and seventy-five thousand. Even the alley is crowded out. Through dark hallways and filthy cellars, crowded, as is every foot of the street, with dirty children, the settlements in the rear are reached. Thieves know how to find them when pursued by the police, and the tramps that sneak in on chilly nights to fight for the warm spot in the yard over some baker's oven. They are out of place in this hive of busy industry, and they know it. It has nothing in common with them or with their philosophy of life, that the world owes the idler a living. Life here means the hardest kind of work almost from the cradle. The world as a debtor has no credit in Jewtown. Its promise to pay wouldn't buy one of the old hats that are hawked about Hester Street, unless backed by security representing labor done at lowest market rates. But this army of workers must have bread. It is cheap and filling, and bakeries abound. Wherever they are in the tenements the tramp will skulk in, if he can. There is such a tramps' roost in the rear of a tenement near the lower end of Ludlow Street, that is never without its tenants in winter. By a judicious practice of flopping over on the stone pavement at intervals and thus warming one side at a time, and with an empty box to put the feet in, it is possible to keep reasonably comfortable there even on a rainy night. In summer the yard is the only one in the neighborhood that does not do duty as a public dormitory.

Thrift is the watchword of Jewtown, as of its people the world over. It is at once its strength and its fatal weakness, its cardinal virtue and its foul disgrace. Become an over-mastering passion with these people who come here in droves from Eastern Europe to escape persecution, from which freedom could be bought only with gold, it has enslaved them in bondage worse than that from which they fled. Money is their God. Life itself is of little value compared with even the leanest bank account. In no other spot does life wear so intensely bald and materialistic an aspect as in Ludlow Street. Over and over again I have met with instances of these Polish or Russian Jews deliberately starving themselves to the point of physical exhaustion, while working night and day at a tremendous pressure to save a little money. An avenging Nemesis pursues this headlong hunt for wealth; there is no worse paid class anywhere. I once put the question to one of their own people, who, being a pawnbroker, and an unusually intelligent and charitable one, certainly enjoyed the advantage of a practical view of the situation: "Whence the many wretchedly poor people in such a colony of workers, where poverty, from a misfortune, has become a reproach, dreaded as the plague?"

"Immigration," he said, "brings us a lot. In five years it has averaged twenty-five thousand a year, of which more than seventy per cent have stayed in New York. Half of them require and receive aid from the Hebrew Charities from the very start, lest they starve. That is one explanation. There is another class than the one that cannot get work: those who have had too much of it; who have worked and hoarded and lived, crowded together like pigs, on the scantiest fare and the worst to be got, bound to save whatever their earnings, until, worn out, they could work no longer. Then their hoards were soon exhausted. That is their story." And I knew that what he said was true.

Penury and poverty are wedded everywhere to dirt and disease, and Jewtown is no exception. It could not well be otherwise in such crowds, considering especially their low intellectual status. The managers of the Eastern Dispensary, which is in the very heart of their district, told the whole story when they said: "The diseases these people suffer from are not due to intemperance or immorality, but to ignorance, want of suitable food, and the foul air in which they live and work."* The homes of the Hebrew quarter are its workshops also. Reference will be made to the economic conditions under which they work in a succeeding chapter. Here we are concerned simply with the fact. You are made fully aware of it before you have travelled the length of a single block in any of these East Side streets, by the whir of a thousand sewing-machines, worked at high pressure from earliest dawn till mind and muscle give out together. Every member of the family, from the youngest to the oldest, bears a hand, shut in the qualmy rooms, where meals are cooked and clothing washed and dried besides, the live-long day. It is not unusual to find a dozen persons—men, women, and children—at work in a single small room. The fact accounts for the contrast that strikes with wonder the observer who comes across from the Bend. Over there the entire population seems possessed of an uncontrollable impulse to get out into the street; here all its energies appear to be bent upon keeping in and away from it. Not that the streets are deserted. The overflow from these tenements is enough to make a crowd anywhere. The children alone would do it. Not old enough to work and no room for play, that is their story. In the home the child's place is usurped by the lodger, who performs the service of the Irishman's pig—pays the rent. In the street the army of hucksters crowd him out. Typhus fever and small-pox are bred here, and help solve the question what to do with him. Filth diseases both, they sprout naturally among the hordes that bring the germs with them from across the sea, and whose first instinct is to hide their sick lest the authorities carry them off to the hospital to be slaughtered, as they firmly believe. The health officers are on constant and sharp lookout for hidden fever-nests. Considering that half of the ready-made clothes that are sold in the big stores, if not a good deal more than half, are made in these tenement rooms, this is not excessive caution. It has happened more than once that a child recovering from small-pox, and in the most contagious stage of the disease, has been found crawling among heaps of half-finished clothing that the next day would be offered for sale on the counter of a Broadway store; or that a typhus fever patient has been discovered in a room whence

* Report of Eastern Dispensary for 1889.

100

perhaps a hundred coats had been sent home that week, each one with the wearer's death-warrant, unseen and unsuspected, basted in the lining.

The health officers call the Tenth the typhus ward; in the office where deaths are registered it passes as the "suicide ward," for reasons not hard to understand; and among the police as the "crooked ward," on account of the number of "crooks," petty thieves and their allies, the "fences," receivers of stolen goods, who find the dense crowds congenial. The nearness of the Bowery, the great "thieves' highway," helps to keep up the supply of these, but Jewtown does not support its dives. Its troubles with the police are the characteristic crop of its intense business rivalries. Oppression, persecution, have not shorn the Jew of his native combativeness one whit. He is as ready to fight for his rights, or what he considers his rights, in a business transaction— synonymous generally with his advantage—as if he had not been robbed of them for eighteen hundred years. One strong impression survives with him from his days of bondage: the power of the law. On the slightest provocation he rushes off to invoke it for his protection. Doubtless the sensation is novel to him, and therefore pleasing. The police at the Eldridge Street station are in a constant turmoil over these everlasting fights. Somebody is always denouncing somebody else, and getting his enemy or himself locked up; frequently both, for the prisoner, when brought in, has generally as plausible a story to tell as his accuser, and as hot a charge to make. The day closes on a wild conflict of rival interests. Another dawns with the prisoner in court, but no complainant. Over night the case has been settled on a business basis, and the police dismiss their prisoner in deep disgust.

These quarrels have sometimes a comic aspect. Thus, with the numerous dancing-schools that are scattered among the synagogues, often keeping them company in the same tenement. They are generally kept by some man who works in the daytime at tailoring, cigarmaking, or something else. The young people in Jewtown are inordinately fond of dancing, and after their day's hard work will flock to these "schools" for a night's recreation. But even to their fun they carry their business preferences, and it happens that a school adjourns in a body to make a general raid

101

on the rival establishment across the street, without the ceremony of paying the admission fee. Then the dance breaks up in a general fight, in which, likely enough, someone is badly hurt. The police come in, as usual, and ring down the curtain.

Bitter as are his private feuds, it is not until his religious life is invaded that a real inside view is obtained of this Jew, whom the history of Christian civilization has taught nothing but fear and hatred. There are two or three missions in the district conducting a hopeless propagandism for the Messiah whom the Tenth Ward rejects, and they attract occasional crowds, who come to hear the Christian preacher as the Jews of old gathered to hear the apostles expound the new doctrine. The result is often strikingly similar. "For once," said a certain well-known minister of an uptown church to me, after such an experience, "I felt justified in comparing myself to Paul preaching salvation to the Jews. They kept still until I spoke of Jesus Christ as the Son of God. Then they got up and fell to arguing among themselves and to threatening me, until it looked as if they meant to take me out in Hester Street and stone me." As at Jerusalem, the Chief Captain was happily at hand with his centurions, in the person of a sergeant and three policemen, and the preacher was rescued. So, in all matters pertaining to their religious life that tinges all their customs, they stand, these East Side Jews, where the new day that dawned on Calvary left them standing, stubbornly refusing to see the light. A visit to a Jewish house of mourning is like bridging the gap of two thousand years. The inexpressibly sad and sorrowful wail for the dead, as it swells and rises in the hush of all sounds of life, comes back from the ages like a mournful echo of the voice of Rachel "weeping for her children and refusing to be comforted, because they are not."

Attached to many of the synagogues, which among the poorest Jews frequently consist of a scantily furnished room in a rear tenement, with a few wooden stools or benches for the congregation, are Talmudic schools that absorb a share of the growing youth. The school-master is not rarely a man of some attainments who has been stranded there, his native instinct for money-making having been smothered in the process that has made of him a learned man. It was of such a school in Eldridge Street that the wicked Isaac Iacob, who killed his enemy, his wife, and himself in one day, was janitor. But the majority of the children seek the public schools, where they are received sometimes with some misgivings on the part of the teachers, who find it necessary to inculcate lessons of cleanliness in the worst cases by practical demonstration with wash-bowl and soap. "He took hold of the soap as if it were some animal," said one of these teachers to me after such an experiment upon a new pupil, "and wiped three fingers across his face. He called that washing." In the Allen Street public school the experienced principal has embodied among the elementary lessons, to keep constantly before the children the duty that clearly lies next to their hands, a characteristic exercise. The question is asked daily from the teacher's desk: "What must I do to be healthy?" and the school responds:

> I must keep my skin clean,
> Wear clean clothes,
> Breathe pure air,
> And live in the sunlight.

It seems little less than biting sarcasm to hear them say it, for to not a few of them all these things are known only by name. In their everyday life there is nothing even to suggest any of them. Only the demand of religious custom has power to make their parents clean up at stated intervals, and the young naturally are no better. As scholars, the children of the most ignorant Polish Jew keep fairly abreast of their more favored playmates, until it comes to mental arithmetic, when they leave them behind with a bound. It is surprising to see how strong the instinct of dollars and cents is in them. They can count, and correctly, almost before they can talk.

Within a few years the police captured on the East Side a band of firebugs who made a business of setting fire to tenements for the insurance on their furniture. There has, unfortunately, been some evidence in the past year that another such conspiracy is on foot. The danger to which these fiends expose their fellow-tenants is appalling. A fire-panic at night in a tenement, by no means among the rare experiences in New York, with the surging, half-

103

smothered crowds on stairs and fire-escapes, the frantic mothers and crying children, the wild struggle to save the little that is their all, is a horror that has few parallels in human experience.

I cannot think without a shudder of one such scene in a First Avenue tenement. It was in the middle of the night. The fire had swept up with sudden fury from a restaurant on the street floor, cutting off escape. Men and women threw themselves from the windows, or were carried down senseless by the firemen. Thirteen half-clad, apparently lifeless bodies were laid on the floor of an adjoining coal-office, and the ambulance surgeons worked over them with sleeves rolled up to the elbows. A half-grown girl with a baby in her arms walked about among the dead and dying with a stunned, vacant look, singing in a low, scared voice to the child. One of the doctors took her arm to lead her out, and patted the cheek of the baby soothingly. It was cold. The baby had been smothered with its father and mother; but the girl, her sister, did not know it. Her reason had fled.

Thursday night and Friday morning are bargain days in the "Pig-market." Then is the time to study the ways of this peculiar people to the best advantage. A common pulse beats in the quarters of the Polish Jews and in the Mulberry Bend, though they have little else in common. Life over yonder in fine weather is a perpetual holiday, here a veritable tread-mill of industry. Friday brings out all the latent color and picturesqueness of the Italians, as of these Semites. The crowds and the common poverty are the bonds of sympathy between them. The Pig-market is in Hester Street, extending either way from Ludlow Street, and up and down the side streets two or three blocks, as the state of trade demands. The name was given to it probably in derision, for pork is the one ware that is not on sale in the Pig-market. There is scarcely anything else that can be hawked from a wagon that is not to be found, and at ridiculously low prices. Bandannas and tin cups at two cents, peaches at a cent a quart, "damaged" eggs for a song, hats for a quarter, and spectacles, warranted to suit the eye, at the optician's who has opened shop on a Hester Street door-step, for thirty-five cents; frowsy-looking chickens and half-plucked geese, hung by the neck and protesting with wildly strutting feet even in death against the outrage, are the great staple of the market. Half or a quarter of a chicken can be bought here by those who cannot afford a whole. It took more than ten years of persistent effort on the part of the sanitary authorities to drive the trade in live fowl from the streets to the fowl-market on Gouverneur Slip, where the killing is now done according to Jewish rite by priests detailed for the purpose by the chief rabbi. Since then they have had a characteristic rumpus, that involved the entire Jewish community, over the fees for killing and the mode of collecting them. Here is a woman churning horse-radish on a machine she has chained and padlocked to a tree on the sidewalk, lest someone steal it. Beside her a butcher's stand with cuts at prices the avenues never dreamed of. Old coats are hawked for fifty cents, "as good as new," and "pants"—there are no trousers in Jewtown, only pants—at anything that can be got. There is a knot of half a dozen "pants" pedlars in the middle of the street, twice as many men of their own race fingering their wares and plucking at the seams with the anxious scrutiny of would-be buyers, though none of them has the least idea of investing in a pair. Yes, stop! This baker, fresh from his trough, bare-headed and with bare arms, has made an offer: for this pair thirty cents; a dollar and forty was the price asked. The pedlar shrugs his shoulders, and turns up his hands with a half pitying, wholly indignant air. What does the baker take him for? Such pants. . . . The baker has turned to go. With a jump like a panther's, the man with the pants has him by the sleeve. Will he give eighty cents? Sixty? Fifty? So help him, they are dirt cheap at that. Lose, will he, on the trade, lose all the profit of his day's peddling. The baker goes on unmoved. Forty then? What, not forty? Take them then for thirty, and wreck the life of a poor man. And the baker takes them and goes, well knowing that at least twenty cents of the thirty, two hundred per cent, were clear profit, if indeed the "pants" cost the pedlar anything.

The suspender pedlar is the mystery of the Pig-market, omni-present and unfathomable. He is met at every step with his wares dangling over his shoulder, down his back, and in front. Millions of suspenders thus perambulate Jewtown all day on a sort of dress parade. Why suspenders, is the puzzle, and where do they all go to? The "pants" of Jewtown hang down with a common

105

accord, as if they had never known the support of suspenders. It appears to be as characteristic a trait of the race as the long beard and the Sabbath silk hat of ancient pedigree. I have asked again and again. No one has ever been able to tell me what becomes of the suspenders of Jewtown. Perhaps they are hung up as bric-à-brac in its homes, or laid away and saved up as the equivalent of cash. I cannot tell. I only know that more suspenders are hawked about the Pig-market every day than would supply the whole of New York for a year, were they all bought and turned to use.

The crowds that jostle each other at the wagons and about the sidewalk shops, where a gutter plank on two ash-barrels does duty for a counter! Pushing, struggling, babbling, and shouting in foreign tongues, a veritable Babel of confusion. An English word falls upon the ear almost with a sense of shock, as something unexpected and strange. In the midst of it all there is a sudden wild scattering, a hustling of things from the street into dark cellars, into backyards and by-ways, a slamming and locking of doors hidden under the improvised shelves and counters. The health officers' cart is coming down the street, preceded and followed by stalwart policemen, who shovel up with scant ceremony the eatables—musty bread, decayed fish and stale vegetables—indifferent to the curses that are showered on them from stoops and windows, and carry them off to the dump. In the wake of the wagon, as it makes its way to the East River after the raid, follow a line of despoiled hucksters shouting defiance from a safe distance. Their clamor dies away with the noise of the market. The endless panorama of the tenements, rows upon rows, between stony streets, stretches to the north, to the south, and to the west as far as the eye reaches.

The Children of the Poor

If the sightseer finds less to engage his interest in Jewtown than in the Bend, outside of the clamoring crowds in the Chasir—the Pig-market—he will discover enough to enlist his sympathies, provided he did not leave them behind when he crossed the Bowery. The loss is his own then. There is that in the desolation of child life in those teeming hives to make the shrivelled heart ache with compassion for its kind and throb with a new life of pain, enough to dispel some prejudices that are as old as our faith, and sometimes, I fear, a good deal stronger. The Russian exile adds to the offence of being an alien and a disturber of economic balances the worse one of being a Jew. Let those who cannot forgive this damaging fact possess their souls in patience. There is some evidence that the welcome he has received in those East Side tenements has done more than centuries of persecution could toward making him forget it himself.

The Italian who comes here gravitates naturally to the oldest and most dilapidated tenements in search of cheap rents, which he doesn't find. The Jew has another plan, characteristic of the man. He seeks out the biggest ones and makes the rent come within his means by taking in boarders, "sweating" his flat to the point of police intervention. That that point is a long way beyond human decency, let alone comfort, an instance from Ludlow Street, that came to my notice while writing this, quite clearly demonstrates. The offender was a tailor, who lived with his wife, two children, and two boarders in two rooms on the top floor. (It

Chapter from *The Children of the Poor* by Jacob Riis, published by Scribner's, New York, 1892.

is always the top floor; in fifteen years of active service as a police reporter I have had to climb to the top floor five times for every one my business was further down, irrespective of where the tenement was or what kind of people lived in it. Crime, suicide, and police business generally seem to bear the same relation to the stairs in a tenement that they bear to poverty itself. The more stairs the more trouble. The deepest poverty is at home in the attic.) But this tailor; with his immediate household, including the boarders, he occupied the larger of the two rooms. The other, a bedroom eight feet square, he sublet to a second tailor and his wife: which couple, following his example as their opportunities allowed, divided the bedroom in two by hanging a curtain in the middle, took one-half for themselves and let the other half to still another tailor with a wife and child. A midnight inspection by the sanitary police was followed by the arrest of the housekeeper and the original tailor, and they were fined or warned in the police-court, I forget which. It doesn't much matter. That the real point was missed was shown by the appearance of the owner of the house, a woman, at Sanitary Headquarters, on the day following, with the charge against the policeman that he was robbing her of her tenants.

The story of inhuman packing of human swarms, of bitter poverty, of landlord greed, of sweater slavery, of darkness and squalor and misery, which these tenements have to tell, is equalled, I suppose, nowhere in a civilized land. Despite the prevalence of the boarder, who is usually a married man, come over alone the better to be able to prepare the way for the family, the census* shows that fifty-four per cent of the entire population of immigrant Jews were children, or under age. Every steamer has added to their number since, and judging from the sights one sees daily in the office of the United Hebrew Charities, and from the general appearance of Ludlow Street, the proportion of children has suffered no decrease. Let the reader who would know for himself what they are like, and what their chances are, take that street some evening from Hester Street down and observe what he sees going on there. Not that it is the only place where he

* The census referred to in this chapter was taken for a special purpose, by a committee of prominent Hebrews, in August, 1890, and was very searching.

can find them. The census I spoke of embraced forty-five streets in the Seventh, Tenth, and Thirteenth Wards. But at that end of Ludlow Street the tenements are taller and the crowds always denser than anywhere else. Let him watch the little pedlars hawking their shoe-strings, their matches, and their penny paper-pads, with the restless energy that seems so strangely out of proportion to the reward it reaps; the half-grown children staggering under heavy bundles of clothes from the sweater's shop; the ragamuffins at their fretful play, play yet, discouraged though it be by the nasty surroundings—thank goodness, every year brings its Passover with the scrubbing brigade to Ludlow Street, and the dirt is shifted from the houses to the streets once anyhow; if it does find its way back, something may be lost on the way—the crowding, the pushing for elbow-room, the wails of bruised babies that keep falling down-stairs, or rolling off the stoop, and the raids of angry mothers swooping down upon their offspring and distributing thumps right and left to pay for the bruises, an eye for an eye, a tooth for a tooth. Whose eye, whose tooth, is of less account in Jewtown than that the capital put out bears awful interest in kind. What kind of interest may society some day expect to reap from Ghettos like these, where even the sunny temper of childhood is soured by want and woe, or smothered in filth? It is a long time since I have heard a good honest laugh, a child's gleeful shout, in Ludlow Street. Angry cries, jeers, enough. They are as much part of the place as the dirty pavements; but joyous, honest laughs, like soap and water, are at a premium there.

But children laugh because they are happy. They are not happy in Ludlow Street. Nobody is except the landlord. Why should they be? Born to toil and trouble, they claim their heritage early and part with it late. There is even less time than there is room for play in Jewtown, good reason why the quality of the play is poor. There is work for the weakest hands, a step for the smallest feet in the vast tread-mill of these East Side homes. A thing is worth there what it will bring. All other considerations, ambitions, desires, yield to that. Education pays as an investment, and therefore the child is sent to school. The moment his immediate value as a worker overbalances the gain in prospect by keeping him at his books, he goes to the shop. The testimony of

109

Jewish observers, who have had quite unusual opportunities for judging, is that the average age at which these children leave school for good is rather below twelve than beyond it, by which time their work at home, helping their parents, has qualified them to earn wages that will more than pay for their keep. They are certainly on the safe side in their reckoning, if the children are not. The legal age for shop employment is fourteen. On my visits among the homes, workshops, and evening schools of Jewtown, I was always struck by the number of diminutive wage-earners who were invariably "just fourteen." It was clearly not the child which the tenement had dwarfed in their case, but the memory or the moral sense of the parents.

If, indeed, the shop were an exchange for the home; if the child quit the one upon entering the other, there might be little objection to make; but too often they are two names for the same thing; where they are not, the shop is probably preferable, bad as that may be. When, in the midnight hour, the noise of the sewing-machine was stilled at last, I have gone the rounds of Ludlow and Hester and Essex Streets among the poorest of the Russian Jews, with the sanitary police, and counted often four, five, and even six of the little ones in a single bed, sometimes a shake-down on the hard floor, often a pile of half-finished clothing brought home from the sweater, in the stuffy rooms of their tenements. In one I visited very lately, the only bed was occupied by the entire family lying lengthwise and crosswise, literally in layers, three children at the feet, all except a boy of ten or twelve, for whom there was no room. He slept with his clothes on to keep him warm, in a pile of rags just inside the door. It seemed to me impossible that families of children could be raised at all in such dens as I had my daily and nightly walks in. And yet the vital statistics and all close observation agree in allotting to these Jews even an unusual degree of good health. The records of the Sanitary Bureau show that while the Italians have the highest death-rate, the mortality in the lower part of the Tenth Ward, of which Ludlow Street is the heart and type, is the lowest in the city. Even the baby death-rate is very low. But for the fact that the ravages of diphtheria, croup, and measles run up the record in the houses occupied entirely by tailors—in other words, in the sweater district, where contagion always runs riot*—the Tenth Ward would seem to be the healthiest spot in the city, as well as the dirtiest and the most crowded. The temperate habits of the Jew and his freedom from enfeebling vices generally must account for this, along with his marvellous vitality. I cannot now recall ever having known a Jewish drunkard. On the other hand, I have never come across a Prohibitionist among them. The absence of the one renders the other superfluous.

It was only last winter I had occasion to visit repeatedly a double tenement at the lower end of Ludlow Street, which the police census showed to contain 297 tenants, 45 of whom were under five years of age, not counting 3 pedlars who slept in the mouldy cellar, where the water was ankle deep on the mud floor. The feeblest ray of daylight never found its way down there, the hatches having been carefully covered with rags and matting; but freshets often did. Sometimes the water rose to the height of a foot, and never quite soaked away in the driest season. It was an awful place, and by the light of my candle the three, with their unkempt beards and hair and sallow faces, looked more like hideous ghosts than living men. Yet they had slept there among and upon decaying fruit and wreckage of all sorts from the tenement for over three years, according to their own and the housekeeper's statements. There had been four. One was then in the hospital, but not because of any ill effect the cellar had had upon him. He had been run over in the street and was making the most of his vacation, charging it up to the owner of the wagon, whom he was getting ready to sue for breaking his leg. Upstairs, especially in the rear tenement, I found the scene from the cellar

---

* Dr. Roger S. Tracy's report of the vital statistics for 1891 shows that, while the general death-rate of the city was 25.96 per 1,000 of the population —that of adults (over five years) 17.13, and the baby death-rate (under five years) 93.21—in the Italian settlement in the west half of the Fourteenth Ward the record stood as follows: general death-rate, 33.52; adult death-rate, 16.29; and baby death-rate, 150.52. In the Italian section of the Fourth Ward it stood: general death-rate, 34.88; adult death-rate, 21.29; baby death-rate, 119.02. In the sweaters' district in the lower part of the Tenth Ward the general death-rate was 16.23; the adult death-rate, 7.59; and the baby death-rate, 61.15. Dr. Tracy adds: "The death-rate from phthisis was highest in houses entirely occupied by cigarmakers (Bohemians), and lowest in those entirely occupied by tailors. On the other hand, the death-rates from diphtheria and croup and measles were highest in houses entirely occupied by tailors."

repeated with variations. In one room a family of seven, including the oldest daughter, a young woman of eighteen, and her brother, a year older than she, slept in a common bed made on the floor of the kitchen, and manifested scarcely any concern at our appearance. A complaint to the Board of Health resulted in an overhauling that showed the tenement to be unusually bad even for that bad spot; but when we came to look up its record, from the standpoint of the vital statistics, we discovered that not only had there not been a single death in the house during the whole year, but on the third floor lived a woman over a hundred years old, who had been there a long time. I was never more surprised in my life, and while we laughed at it, I confess it came nearer to upsetting my faith in the value of statistics than anything I had seen till then. And yet I had met with similar experiences, if not quite so striking, often enough to convince me that poverty and want beget their own power to resist the evil influences of their worst surroundings. I was at a loss how to put this plainly to the good people who often asked wonderingly why the children of the poor one saw in the street seemed generally such a thriving lot, until a slip of Mrs. Partington's discriminating tongue did it for me: "Manured to the soil." That is it. In so far as it does not merely seem so—one does not see the sick and suffering—that puts it right.

Whatever the effect upon the physical health of the children, it cannot be otherwise, of course, than that such conditions should corrupt their morals. I have the authority of a distinguished rabbi, whose field and daily walk are among the poorest of his people, to support me in the statement that the moral tone of the young girls is distinctly lower than it was. The entire absence of privacy in their homes and the foul contact of the sweaters' shops, where men and women work side by side from morning till night, scarcely half clad in the hot summer weather, does for the girls what the street completes in the boy. But for the patriarchal family life of the Jew that is his strongest virtue, their ruin would long since have been complete. It is that which pilots him safely through shoals upon which the Gentile would have been inevitably wrecked. It is that which keeps the almshouse from casting its shadow over Ludlow Street to add to its gloom.

It is the one quality which redeems, and on the Sabbath eve when he gathers his household about his board, scant though the fare be, dignifies the darkest slum of Jewtown.

How strong is this attachment to home and kindred that makes the Jew cling to the humblest hearth and gather his children and his children's children about it, though grinding poverty leave them only a bare crust to share, I saw in the case of little Jette Brodsky, who strayed away from her own door, looking for her papa. They were strangers and ignorant and poor, so that weeks went by before they could make their loss known and get a hearing, and meanwhile Jette, who had been picked up and taken to Police Headquarters, had been hidden away in an asylum, given another name when nobody came to claim her, and had been quite forgotten. But in the two years that passed before she was found at last, her empty chair stood ever by her father's, at the family board, and no Sabbath eve but heard his prayer for the restoration of their lost one. It happened once that I came in on a Friday evening at the breaking of bread, just as the four candles upon the table had been lit with the Sabbath blessing upon the home and all it sheltered. Their light fell on little else than empty plates and anxious faces; but in the patriarchal host who arose and bade the guest welcome with a dignity a king might have envied I recognized with difficulty the humble pedlar I had known only from the street and from the police office, where he hardly ventured beyond the door.

But the tenement that has power to turn purest gold to dross digs a pit for the Jew even through this virtue that has been his shield against its power for evil. In its atmosphere it turns too often to a curse by helping to crowd his lodgings, already over-flowing, beyond the point of official forbearance. Then follow orders to "reduce" the number of tenants that mean increased rent, which the family cannot pay, or the breaking up of the home. An appeal to avert such a calamity came to the Board of Health recently from one of the refuge tenements. The tenant was a man with a houseful of children, too full for the official scale as applied to the flat, and his plea was backed by the influence of his only friend in need—the family undertaker. There was something so cruelly suggestive in the idea that the laugh it raised died without an echo.

113

The census of the sweaters' district gave a total of 23,405 children under six years, and 21,285 between six and fourteen, in a population of something over a hundred and eleven thousand Russian, Polish, and Roumanian Jews in the three wards mentioned; 15,567 are set down as "children over fourteen." According to the record, scarce one-third of the heads of families had become naturalized citizens, though the average of their stay in the United States was between nine and ten years. The very language of our country was to them a strange tongue, understood and spoken by only 15,837 of the fifty thousand and odd adults enumerated. Seven thousand of the rest spoke only German, five thousand Russian, and over twenty-one thousand could only make themselves understood to each other, never to the world around them, in the strange jargon that passes for Hebrew on the East Side, but is really a mixture of a dozen known dialects and tongues and of some that were never known or heard anywhere else. In the census it is down as just what it is—jargon, and nothing else.

Here, then, are conditions as unfavorable to the satisfactory, even safe, development of child life in the chief American city as could well be imagined; more unfavorable even than with the Bohemians, who have at least their faith in common with us, if safety lies in the merging through the rising generation of the discordant elements into a common harmony. A community set apart, set sharply against the rest in every clashing interest, social and industrial; foreign in language, in faith, and in tradition; repaying dislike with distrust; expanding under the new relief from oppression in the unpopular qualities of greed and contentiousness fostered by ages of tyranny unresistingly borne. Clearly, if ever there was need of moulding any material for the citizenship that awaits it, it is with this; and if ever trouble might be expected to beset the effort, it might be looked for here. But it is not so. The record shows that of the sixty thousand children, including the fifteen thousand young men and women over fourteen who earn a large share of the money that pays for rent and food, and the twenty-three thousand toddlers under six years, fully one-third go to school. Deducting the two extremes, little more than a thousand children of between six and fourteen years, that is, of school age, were put down as receiving no instruction at the time the census was taken; but it is not at all likely that this condition was permanent in the case of the greater number of these. The poorest Hebrew knows—the poorer he is, the better he knows it—that knowledge is power, and power as the means of getting on in the world that has spurned him so long is what his soul yearns for. He lets no opportunity slip to obtain it. Day and night schools are crowded by his children, who are everywhere forging ahead of their Christian school-fellows, taking more than their share of prizes and promotions. Every synagogue, every second rear tenement or dark back yard, has its school and its school-master with his scourge to intercept those who might otherwise escape. In the census there are put down 251 Jewish teachers as living in these tenements, a large number of whom conduct such schools, so that, as the children form always more than one-half of the population in the Jewish quarter, the evidence is after all that even here, with the tremendous inpour of a destitute, ignorant people, and with the undoubted employment of child labor on a large scale, the cause of progress along the safe line is holding its own.

It is true that these tenement schools that absorb several thousand children are not what they might be from a sanitary point of view. It is also true that heretofore nothing but Hebrew and the Talmud have been taught there. But to the one evil the health authorities have recently been aroused; of the other, the wise and patriotic men who are managing the Baron de Hirsch charity are making a useful handle by gathering the teachers in and setting them to learn English. Their new knowledge will soon be reflected in their teaching, and the Hebrew schools become primary classes in the system of public education. The school in a Hester Street tenement is a fair specimen of its kind—by no means one of the worst—and so is the backyard behind it, that serves as the children's play-ground, with its dirty mud-puddles, its slop-barrels and broken flags, and its foul tenement-house surroundings. Both fall in well with the home lives and environment of the unhappy little wretches whose daily horizon they limit. They get there the first instruction they receive in the only tongues with which the teachers are familiar, Hebrew and the Jargon, in the only studies which they are competent to teach, the Talmud and the Prophets. Until they are six years old they are under the "Melammed's" rod all day; after that only in the interval between public school and supper. It is practically the only religious instruction the poorest Jewish children receive, but it is claimed by some of their rabbis that they had better have none at all. The daily transition, they say, from the bright and, by comparison, aesthetically beautiful public school-room to these dark and inhospitable dens, with which the faith that has brought so many miseries upon their race comes to be inseparably associated in the child's mind as he grows up, tends to reflections that breed indifference, if not infidelity, in the young. It would not be strange if this were so. If the schools, through this process, also help pave the way for the acceptance of the Messiah heretofore rejected, which I greatly doubt, it may be said to be the only instance in which the East Side tenement has done its tenants a good Christian turn.

There is no more remarkable class in any school than that of these Melammedim,* that may be seen in session any week-day forenoon, save on Saturday, of course, in the Hebrew Institute in East Broadway. Old bearded men struggling through the intricacies of the first reader, "a cow, a cat," and all the rest of childish learning, with a rapt attention and a concentration of energy as if they were devoting themselves to the most heroic of tasks, which, indeed, they are, for the good that may come of it cannot easily be overestimated. As an educational measure it may be said to be getting down to first principles with a vengeance. When the reader has been mastered, brief courses in the history of the United States, the Declaration of Independence, and the Constitution follow. The test of proficiency in the pupil is his ability to translate the books of the Old Testament, with which he is familiar, of course, from Hebrew into English, and *vice versa*. The Melammed is rarely a dull scholar. No one knows better than he, to whom it has come only in the evening of his hard life, the value of the boon that is offered him. One of the odd group that was deep in the lesson of the day had five children at home, whom he had struggled to bring up on an income of ten dollars a week. The oldest, a bright

* Meaning "teachers."

116

boy who had graduated with honor, despite the patch on his trousers, from the public school, was ambitious to go to college, and the father had saved and pinched in a thousand ways to gratify his desire. One of the managers of the Institute who knew how the family were starving on half rations, had offered the father, a short time before, to get the boy employment in a store at three dollars a week. It was a tremendous temptation, for the money was badly needed at home. But the old man put it resolutely away from him. "No," he said, "I must send him to college. He shall have the chance that was denied his father." And he was as good as his word. And so was the lad, a worthy son of a worthy father. When I met him he had already proved himself a long way the best student in his class.

In other class-rooms in the great building, which is devoted entirely to the cause of Americanizing the young Russian immigrants, hundreds of children get daily their first lessons in English and in patriotism in simultaneous doses. The two are inseparable in the beneficent plan of their instructors. Their effort is to lay hold of the children of the new-comers at once; tender years are no barrier. For the toddlers there are kindergarten classes, with play the street has had no chance to soil. And while playing they learn to speak the strange new tongue and to love the pretty flag with the stars that is everywhere in sight. The night school gathers in as many as can be corralled of those who are big enough, if not old enough, to work. The ease and rapidity with which they learn is equalled only by their good behavior and close attention while in school. There is no whispering and no rioting at these desks, no trial of strength with the teacher, as in the Italian ragged schools, where the question who is boss has always to be settled before the business of the school can proceed. These children come to learn. Even from the Christian schools in the district that gather in their share comes the same testimony. All the disturbance they report was made by their elders, outside the school, in the street. In the Hebrew Institute the average of absence for all causes was, during the first year, less than eight per cent of the registered attendance, and in nearly every case sickness furnished a valid excuse. In a year and a half the principal had only been called upon three times to reprove an obstreperous pupil, in a total of 1,500. While I was

117

visiting one of the day classes a little girl who had come from Moscow only two months before presented herself with her green vaccination card from the steamer. She understood already perfectly the questions put to her and was able to answer most of them in English. Boys of eight and nine years who had come over as many months before, knowing only the jargon of their native village, read to me whole pages from the reader with almost perfect accent, and did sums on the blackboard that would have done credit to the average boy of twelve in our public schools. Figuring is always their strong point. They would not be Jews if it was not.

In the evening classes the girls of "fourteen" flourished, as everywhere in Jewtown. There were many who were much older, and some who were a long way yet from that safe goal. One sober-faced little girl, who wore a medal for faithful attendance and who could not have been much over ten, if as old as that, said that she "went out dressmaking" and so helped her mother. Another, who was even smaller and had been here just three weeks, yet understood what was said to her, explained in broken German that she was learning to work at "Blumen" in a Grand Street shop, and would soon be able to earn wages that would help support the family of four children, of whom she was the oldest. The girl who sat in the seat with her was from a Hester Street tenement. Her clothes showed that she was very poor. She read very fluently on demand a story about a big dog that tried to run away, or something, "when he had a chance." When she came to translate what she had read into German, which many of the Russian children understand, she got along until she reached the word "chance." There she stopped, bewildered. It was the one idea of which her brief life had no embodiment, the thing it had altogether missed.

The Declaration of Independence half the children knew by heart before they had gone over it twice. To help them along it is printed in the school-books with a Hebrew translation and another in Jargon, a "Jewish-German," in parallel columns and the explanatory notes in Hebrew. The Constitution of the United States is treated in the same manner, but it is too hard, or too wearisome, for the children. They "hate" it, says the teacher, while the Declaration of Independence takes their fancy at sight.

They understand it in their own practical way, and the spirit of the immortal document suffers no loss from the annotations of Ludlow Street, if its dignity is sometimes slightly rumpled.

"When," said the teacher to one of the pupils, a little working-girl from an Essex Street sweater's shop, "the Americans could no longer put up with the abuse of the English who governed the colonies, what occurred then?"

"A strike!" responded the girl, promptly. She had found it here on coming and evidently thought it a national institution upon which the whole scheme of our government was founded.

It was curious to find the low voices of the children, particularly the girls, an impediment to instruction in this school. They could sometimes hardly be heard for the noise in the street, when the heat made it necessary to have the windows open. But shrillness is not characteristic even of the Pig-market when it is noisiest and most crowded. Some of the children had sweet singing voices. One especially, a boy with straight red hair and a freckled face, chanted in a plaintive minor key the One Hundred and Thirtieth Psalm, "Out of the depths" etc., and the harsh gutturals of the Hebrew became sweet harmony until the sad strain brought tears to our eyes.

*   *   *   *   *   *   *

The smoky torches on many hucksters' carts threw their uncertain yellow light over Hester Street as I watched the children troop homeward from school one night. Eight little pedlars hawking their wares had stopped under the lamp on the corner to bargain with each other for want of cash customers. They were engaged in a desperate but vain attempt to cheat one of their number who was deaf and dumb. I bought a quire of note-paper of the mute for a cent and instantly the whole crew beset me in a fierce rivalry, to which I put a hasty end by buying out the little mute's poor stock—ten cents covered it all—and after he had counted out the quires, gave it back to him. At this act of unheard-of generosity the seven, who had remained to witness the transfer, stood speechless. As I went my way, with a sudden common impulse they kissed their hands at me, all rivalry forgotten in their admiration, and kept kissing, bowing, and salaaming

119

until I was out of sight. "Not bad children," I mused as I went along, "good stuff in them, whatever their faults." I thought of the poor boy's stock, of the cheapness of it, and then it occurred to me that he had charged me just twice as much for the paper I gave him back as for the penny quire I bought. But when I went back to give him a piece of my mind the boys were gone.

My Ten Years' War with the Slums

In a Stanton Street tenement, the other day, I stumbled upon a Polish capmaker's home. There were other capmakers in the house, Russian and Polish, but they simply "lived" there. This one had a home. The fact proclaimed itself the moment the door was opened, in spite of the darkness. The rooms were in the rear, gloomy with the twilight of the tenement, although the day was sunny without, but neat, even cosy. It was early, but the day's chores were evidently done. The teakettle sang on the stove, at which a bright-looking girl of twelve, with a pale but cheery face, and sleeves brushed back to the elbows, was busy poking up the fire. A little boy stood by the window, flattening his nose against the pane and gazing wistfully up among the chimney pots where a piece of blue sky about as big as the kitchen could be made out. I remarked to the mother that they were nice rooms.

"Ah yes," she said, with a weary little smile that struggled bravely with hope long deferred, "but it is hard to make a home here. We would so like to live in the front, but we can't pay the rent."

I knew the front with its unlovely view of the tenement street too well, and I said a good word for the air shaft—yard or court it could not be called, it was too small for that—which rather surprised myself. I had found few virtues enough in it before. The girl at the stove had left off poking the fire. She broke in the moment I finished, with eager enthusiasm: "Why, they have the sun in there. When the door is opened the light comes right in your face."

Selection from Jacob Riis's *My Ten Years' War with the Slums*, published by Houghton Mifflin Company, Boston, 1900.

"Does it never come here?" I asked, and wished I had not done so, as soon as the words were spoken. The child at the window was listening, with his whole hungry little soul in his eyes.

Yes, it did, she said. Once every summer, for a little while, it came over the houses. She knew the month and the exact hour of the day when its rays shone into their home, and just the reach of its slant on the wall. They had lived there six years. In June the sun was due. A haunting fear that the baby would ask how long it was till June—it was February then—took possession of me, and I hastened to change the subject. Warsaw was their old home. They kept a little store there, and were young and happy. Oh, it was a fine city, with parks and squares, and bridges over the beautiful river—and grass and flowers and birds and soldiers, put in the girl breathlessly. She remembered. But the children kept coming, and they went across the sea to give them a better chance. Father made fifteen dollars a week, much money; but there were long seasons when there was no work. She, the mother, was never very well here—she hadn't any strength; and the baby! She glanced at his grave white face, and took him in her arms. The picture of the two, and of the pale-faced girl longing back to the fields and the sunlight, in their prison of gloom and gray walls, haunts me yet. I have not had the courage to go back since. I recalled the report of an English army surgeon, which I read years ago, on the many more soldiers that died—were killed would be more correct—in barracks into which the sun never shone than in those that were open to the light.

The capmaker's case is the case of the nineteenth century, of civilization, against the metropolis of America. The home, the family, are the rallying points of civilization. But long since the tenements of New York earned for it the ominous name of "the homeless city." In its 40,000 tenements its workers, more than half of the city's population, are housed. They have no other chance. There are, indeed, wives and mothers who, by sheer force of character, rise above their environment and make homes where they go. Happily, there are yet many of them. But the fact remains that hitherto their struggle has been growing ever harder, and the issue more doubtful.

122

The tenement itself, with its crowds, its lack of privacy, is the greatest destroyer of individuality, of character. As its numbers increase, so does "the element that becomes criminal for lack of individuality and the self-respect that comes with it." Add the shiftless and the weak who are turned out by the same process, and you have its legitimate crop. In 1880 the average number of persons to each dwelling in New York was 16.37; in 1890 it was 18.52. In 1895, according to the police census, 21.2. The census of 1900 will show the crowding to have gone on at an equal if not at a greater rate. That will mean that so many more tenements have been built of the modern type, with four families to the floor where once there were two. I shall not weary the reader with many statistics. They are to be found, by those who want them, in the census books and in the official records. I shall try to draw from them their human story. But, as an instance of the unchecked drift, let me quote here the case of the Tenth Ward, that East Side district known as the most crowded in all the world. In 1880, when it had not yet attained that bad eminence, it contained 47,554 persons, or 432.3 to the acre. In 1890 the census showed a population of 57,596, which was 522 to the acre. The police census of 1895 found 70,168 persons living in 1514 houses, which was 643.80 to the acre. Lastly, the Health Department's census for the first half of 1898 gave a total of 82,175 persons living in 1201 tenements, with 313 inhabited buildings yet to be heard from. This is the process of doubling up—literally, since the cause and the vehicle of it all is the double-decker tenement—which in the year 1895 had crowded a single block in that ward at the rate of 1526 persons per acre, and one in the Eleventh Ward at the rate of 1774.* It goes on not in the Tenth Ward or on the East Side only, but throughout the city. When, in 1897, it was proposed to lay out a small park in the Twenty-Second Ward, up on the far West Side, it was shown that five blocks in that section, between Forty-Ninth and Sixty-Second streets and Ninth and Eleventh avenues, had a population of more than 3000 each. The block between Sixty-First

* Police census of 1895: Block bounded by Canal, Hester, Eldridge, and Forsyth streets: size 375 × 200, population 2628, rate per acre 1526. Block bounded by Stanton, Houston, Attorney, and Ridge streets: size 200 × 300, population 2244, rate per acre 1774.

and Sixty-Second streets, Tenth and Eleventh avenues, harbored 3580, which meant 974.6 persons to the acre.

If we have here to do with forces that are beyond the control of the individual or the community, we shall do well at least to face the facts squarely and know the truth. It is no answer to the charge that New York's way of housing its workers is the worst in the world to say that they are better off than they were where they came from. It is not true, in most cases, as far as the home is concerned: a shanty is better than a flat in a cheap tenement, any day. Even if it were true, it would still be beside the issue. In Poland my capmaker counted for nothing. Nothing was expected of him. Here he ranks, after a few brief years, politically equal with the man who hires his labor. A citizen's duty is expected of him, and home and citizenship are convertible terms. The observation of the Frenchman who had watched the experiment of herding two thousand human beings in eight tenement barracks in Paris, that the result was the "exasperation of the tenant against society," is true the world over. We have done as badly in New York. Social hatefulness is not a good soil for citizenship to grow in, where political equality rules.

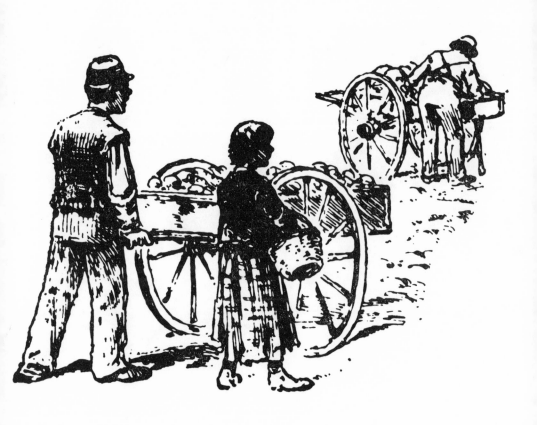

HUTCHINS HAPGOOD

Hutchins Hapgood was born of New England and New York parents in the city of Chicago on May 21, 1869. He was feared lost for a time with his nurse in the great fire of 1871. He received his A.B. degree from the University of Michigan and then went on to an M.A. degree at Harvard, where he taught for a year. He also taught at the University of Chicago, but felt himself strongly drawn toward a more active journalistic life and joined the staff of the reorganized New York *Commercial Advertiser* under the editorship of Lincoln Steffens in 1897. He married Neith Bayes, who wrote for the same paper, in 1899 and had two daughters and two sons with her.

His wide-ranging travels had begun as early as 1893 when he made a trip around the world and resided briefly in Japan. In addition to the *Commercial Advertiser,* he also worked for the *New York Evening Post,* the *New York Telegraph,* the *Chicago Evening Post,* and the *New York Globe,* where he did his most important signed and unsigned newspaper articles. He wrote for magazines, too (some of the chapters of *The Spirit of the Ghetto* appeared first in leading magazines of his day), and delivered public lectures.

Looking back upon his work, Hapgood wrote: "I consider the general character of my work an interpretation of the developing labor, sociological, philosophical, and aesthetic movements of the country. The readers of my autobiography will see how closely I have been connected with almost all the 'movements' of the last forty years. My attitude of mind has consistently been what is

127

called progressive. Sometimes I have been known as a radical, but I think those who best understand me feel that mine was a consistent effort to interpret the developing movements of all kinds." This was written in reply to questions from the editors of the reference work *Twentieth Century Authors*. In the autobiography to which he refers, called *A Victorian in the Modern World*, Hapgood has some penetrating things to say about his own attitudes and motivations: "[I have been] unwilling to accept the standards of value existing among 'the best people' of America. In fact, it is rare that I have met distinguished men and women who have not disappointed me; I have often liked them but they have almost never measured up to their reputation in my feeling. On the other hand, those people who are regarded as evil, or unworthy, have often had for me a strange and haunting appeal. And, indeed, it is through them that my purely personal and temperamental interest in things of social, as contrasted with 'society,' importance had its origin."

It is to this source that we must trace not only *The Spirit of the Ghetto* but such books of his as *The Autobiography of a Thief, An Anarchist Woman,* and *The Spirit of Labor*. In an article paying tribute to Hapgood in the pages of the *New Republic*, his friend Robert Morss Lovett wrote as follows: "His approach to the labor movement is that of an idealist, with a sense of the ultimate values to be released for all mankind when the revolution shall have accomplished its purpose. His interest in the underdog, and belief that unappreciated values lie hidden in the outcast, first animated his study of criminal life; and his *Autobiography of a Thief* was the product of a long and intimate connection with the hero. Later he came to believe that crime was relatively unimportant; and his desire to make the good life possible for the greatest exploited section of society brought him to write *The Spirit of Labor*. In most of his books he maintained the plan of entering heart and soul into the experience of a typical character, and producing what he called 'assisted biography' on the model of *Moll Flanders*."

During most of his life his brother Norman Hapgood was better known than he was, but since his death on November 8, 1944, it is Hutchins Hapgood's work (mostly because of the importance of the subject matter which he chose) which has kept the family name in the light of public attention. His obituary in the *New York Times* recognized his contribution as "a leader in liberal literary circles a quarter of a century ago and in the movements which gave birth to the Greenwich Village tradition and the artists' Provincetown. . . . Mr. Hapgood was among the first to explore the artistic, literary and human riches of New York's East Side. He helped to organize the Provincetown Theater, wrote for it and even acted for it."

Robert Morss Lovett, who has already been quoted, remarked: "For many years in America and parts of Europe it has been an open sesame to say 'Friend of Hutchins Hapgood.'" More critical are the authors of a book called *Rebel America: The Story of Social Revolt in the United States* (1934) in which Hapgood is described ironically as a "product of respectability and Harvard [who] was naively fascinated by the hardboiled Rabelaisian Johannsen, who was later to figure in the McNamara affair, and by the 'free souled' but essentially sentimental posturings of the 'fallen woman' gone intellectual."

Hapgood's limitations are obvious, yet, despite his handicaps, he succeeded in producing some work which has not altogether lost its interest and value for us today.

The Spirit of the Ghetto

A ragged man, who looks like a peddler or a beggar, picking his way through the crowded misery of Hester Street, or ascending the stairs of one of the dingy tenement houses full of sweat-shops that line that busy mart of the poor Ghetto Jew, may be a great Hebrew scholar. He may be able to speak and write the ancient tongue with the facility of a modern language—as fluently as the ordinary Jew makes use of the "jargon," the Yiddish of the people; he may be a manifold author with a deep and pious love for the beautiful poetry in his literature; and in character an enthusiast, a dreamer, or a good and reverend old man. But no matter what his attainments and his quality he is unknown and unhonored, for he has pinned his faith to a declining cause, writes his passionate accents in a tongue more and more unknown even to the cultivated Jew; and consequently amid the crowding and material interests of the new world he is submerged—poor in physical estate and his moral capital unrecognized by the people among whom he lives.

Not only unrecognized by the ignorant and the busy and their teachers, the rabbis, who in New York are frequently nearly as ignorant as the people, he is also (as his learning is limited largely to the literature of his race) looked down upon by the influential and intellectual element of the Ghetto—an element socialistic, in literary sympathy Russian rather than Hebraic, intolerant of everything not violently modern, wedded to "movements" and scornful of the past. The "maskil," therefore, or "man

Selections from *The Spirit of the Ghetto* by Hutchins Hapgood, published by Funk and Wagnalls, New York, 1902.

130

of wisdom"—the Hebrew scholar—is called "old fogy," or "dilettante," by the up-to-date socialists.

Of such men there are several in the humble corners of the New York Ghetto. One peddles for a living, another has a small printing-office in a basement on Canal Street, a third occasionally tutors in some one of many languages and sells a patent medicine, and a fourth is the principal of the Talmud-Thora, a Hebrew school in the Harlem Ghetto, where he teaches the children to read, write, and pray in the Hebrew language.

Moses Reicherson is the name of the principal. "Man of wisdom" of the purest kind, probably the finest Hebrew grammarian in New York, and one of the finest in the world, his income from his position at the head of the school is $5 a week. He is seventy-three years old, wears a thick gray beard, a little cap on his head, and a long black coat. His wife is old and bent. They are alone in their miserable little apartment on East One Hundred and Sixth Street. Their son died a year or two ago, and to cover the funeral expenses Mr. Reicherson tried in vain to sell his "Encyclopædia Britannica." But, nevertheless, the old scholar, who had been bending over his closely written manuscript, received the visitor with almost cheerful politeness, and told the story of his work and of his ambitions. Of his difficulties and privations he said little, but they shone through his words and in the character of the room in which he lived.

Born in Vilna, sometimes called the Jerusalem of Lithuania or the Athens of modern Judæa because of the number of enlightened Jews who have been born there, many of whom now live in the Russian Jewish quarter of New York, he has retained the faith of his orthodox parents, a faith, however, springing from the pure origin of Judaism rather than holding to the hair-splitting distinctions later embodied in the Talmud. He was a teacher of Hebrew in his native town for many years, where he stayed until he came to New York some years ago to be near his son. His two great intellectual interests, subordinated indeed to the love of the old literature and religion, have been Hebrew grammar and the moral fables of several languages. On the former he has written an important work, and of the latter has translated much of Lessing's and Gellert's work into pure Hebrew. He has also translated into his favorite tongue the Russian fable-writer Krilow; has written fables of his own, and a Hebrew commentary on the Bible in twenty-four volumes. He loves the fables "because they teach the people and are real criticism; they are profound and combine fancy and thought." Many of these are still in manuscript, which is characteristic of much of the work of these scholars, for they have no money, and publishers do not run after Hebrew books. Also unpublished, written in lovingly minute characters, he has a Hebrew prayer-book in many volumes. He has written hundreds of articles for the Hebrew weeklies and monthlies, which are fairly numerous in this country, but which seldom can afford to pay their contributors. At present he writes exclusively for a Hebrew weekly published in Chicago, *Regeneration,* the object of which is to promote "the knowledge of the ancient Hebrew language and literature, and to regenerate the spirit of the nation." For this he receives no pay, the editor being almost as poor as himself. But he writes willingly for the love of the cause, "for universal good"; for Reicherson, in common with the other neglected scholars, is deeply interested in revivifying what is now among American Jews a dead language. He believes that in this way only can the Jewish people be taught the good and the true.

"When the national language and literature live," he said, "the nation lives; when dead, so is the nation. The holy tongue in which the Bible was written must not die. If it should, much of the truth of the Bible, many of its spiritual secrets, much of its beautiful poetry, would be lost. I have gone deep into the Bible, that greatest book, all my life, and I know many of its secrets." He beamed with pride as he said these words, and his sense of the beauty of the Hebrew spirit and the Hebrew literature led him to speak wonderingly of anti-Semitism. This cause seemed to him to be founded on ignorance of the Bible. "If the anti-Semites would only study the Bible, would go deep into the knowledge of Hebrew and the teaching of Christ, then everything would be sweet and well. If they would spend a little of that money in supporting the Hebrew language and literature and explaining the sacred books which they now use against our race, they would see that they are anti-Christians rather than anti-Semites."

The scholar here bethought himself of an old fable he had

translated into Hebrew. Cold and Warmth make a wager that the traveller will unwrap his cloak sooner to one than to the other. The fierce wind tries its best, but at every cold blast the traveller only wraps his cloak the closer. But when the sun throws its rays the wayfarer gratefully opens his breast to the warming beams. "Love solves all things," said the old man, "and hate closes up the channels to knowledge and virtue." Believing the Pope to be a good man with a knowledge of the Bible, he wanted to write him about the anti-Semites, but desisted on the reflection that the Pope was very old and overburdened, and that the letter would probably fall into the hands of the cardinals.

All this was sweetly said, for about him there was nothing of the attitude of complaint. His wife once or twice during the interview touched upon their personal condition, but her husband severely kept his mind on the universal truths, and only when questioned admitted that he would like a little more money, in order to publish his books and to enable him to think with more concentration about the Hebrew language and literature. There was no bitterness in his reference to the neglect of Hebrew scholarship in the Ghetto. His interest was impersonal and detached, and his regret at the decadence of the language seemed noble and disinterested; and, unlike some of the other scholars, the touch of warm humanity was in everything he said. Indeed, he is rather the learned teacher of the people with deep religious and ethical sense than the scholar who cares only for learning. "In the name of God, adieu!" he said, with quiet intensity when the visitor withdrew.

Contrasting sharply in many respects with this beautiful old teacher is the man who peddles from tenement house to tenement house in the downtown Ghetto, to support himself and his three young children. S. B. Schwartzberg, unlike most of the "submerged" scholars, is still a young man, only thirty-seven years old, but he is already discouraged, bitter, and discontented. He feels himself the apostle of a lost cause—the regeneration in New York of the old Hebrew language and literature. His great enterprise in life has failed. He has now given it up, and the natural vividness and intensity of his nature get satisfaction in the strenuous abuse of the Jews of the Ghetto.

He was born in Warsaw, Poland, the son of a distinguished

rabbi. In common with many Russian and Polish Jews, he early obtained a living knowledge of the Hebrew language, and a great love of the literature, which he knows thoroughly, altho, unlike Reicherson and a scholar who is to be mentioned, Rosenberg, he has not contributed to the literature in a scientific sense. He is slightly bald, with burning black eyes, an enthusiastic and excited manner, and talks with almost painful earnestness.

Three years ago Schwartzberg came to this country with a great idea in his head. "In this free country," he thought to himself, "where there are so many Russian and Polish Jews, it is a pity that our tongue is dying, is falling into decay, and that the literature and traditions that hold our race together are being undermined by materialism and ethical skepticism." He had a little money, and he decided he would establish a journal in the interests of the Hebrew language and literature. No laws would prevent him here from speaking his mind in his beloved tongue. He would bring into vivid being again the national spirit of his people, make them love with the old fervor their ancient traditions and language. It was the race's spirit of humanity and feeling for the ethical beauty, not the special creed of Judaism, for which he and the other scholars care little, that filled him with the enthusiasm of an apostle. In his monthly magazine, the *Western Light,* he put his best efforts, his best thoughts about ethical truths and literature. The poet Dolitzki contributed in purest Hebrew verse, as did many other Ghetto lights. But it received no support, few bought it, and it lasted only a year. Then he gave it up, bankrupt in money and hope. That was several years ago, and since then he has peddled for a living.

The failure has left in Schwartzberg's soul a passionate hatred of what he calls the materialism of the Jews in America. Only in Europe, he thinks, does the love of the spiritual remain with them. Of the rabbis of the Ghetto he spoke with bitterness. "They," he said, "are the natural teachers of the people. They could do much for the Hebrew literature and language. Why don't they? Because they know no Hebrew and have no culture. In Russia the Jews demand that their rabbis should be learned and spiritual, but here they are ignorant and materialistic." So Mr. Schwartzberg wrote a pamphlet which is now famous in the

134

Ghetto. "I wrote it with my heart's blood," he said, his eyes snapping. "In it I painted the spiritual condition of the Jews in New York in the gloomiest of colors."

"It is terrible," he proceeded vehemently. "Not one Hebrew magazine can exist in this country. They all fail, and yet there are many beautiful Hebrew writers to-day. When Dolitzki was twenty years old in Russia he was looked up to as a great poet. But what do the Jews care about him here? For he writes in Hebrew! Why, Hebrew scholars are regarded by the Jews as tramps, as useless beings. Driven from Russia because we are Jews, we are despised in New York because we are Hebrew scholars! The rabbis, too, despise the learned Hebrew, and they have a fearful influence on the ignorant people. If they can dress well and speak English it is all they want. It is a shame how low-minded these teachers of the people are. I was born of a rabbi, and brought up by him, but in Russia they are for literature and the spirit, while in America it is just the other way."

The discouraged apostle of Hebrew literature now sees no immediate hope for the cause. What seems to him the most beautiful lyric poetry in the world he thinks doomed to the imperfect understanding of generations for whom the language does not live. The only ultimate hope is in the New Jerusalem. Consequently the fiery scholar, altho not a Zionist, thinks well of the movement as tending to bring the Jews again into a nation which shall revive the old tongue and traditions. Mr. Schwartzberg referred to some of the other submerged scholars of the Ghetto. His eyes burned with indignation when he spoke of Moses Reicherson. He could hardly control himself at the thought that the greatest Hebrew grammarian living, "an old man, too, a reverend old man," should be brought to such a pass. In the same strain of outrage he referred to another old man, a scholar who would be as poor as Reicherson and himself were it not for his wife, who is a dressmaker. It is she who keeps him out of the category of "submerged" scholars.

But the Rev. H. Rosenberg, of whose condition Schwartzberg also bitterly complained, is indeed submerged. He runs a printing-office in a Canal Street basement, where he sits in the damp all day long waiting for an opportunity to publish his *magnum opus*, a cyclopedia of Biblical literature, containing an historical and geographical description of the persons, places, and objects mentioned in the Bible. All the Ghetto scholars speak of this work with bated breath, as a tremendously learned affair. Only two volumes of it have been published. To give the remainder to the world, Mr. Rosenberg is waiting for his children, who are nearly self-supporting, to contribute their mite. He is a man of sixty-two, with the high, bald forehead of a scholar. For twenty years he was a rabbi in Russia, and has preached in thirteen synagogues. He has been nine years in New York, and, in addition to the great cyclopedia, has written, but not published, a cyclopedia of Talmudical literature. A *History of the Jews*, in the Russian language, and a Russian novel, *The Jew of Trient*, are among his published works. He is one of the most learned of all of these men who have a living, as well as an exact, knowledge of what is generally regarded as a dead language and literature.

Altho he is waiting to publish the great cyclopedia, he is patient and cold. He has not the sweet enthusiasm of Reicherson, and not the vehement and partisan passion of Schwartzberg. He has the coldness of old age, without its spiritual glow, and scholarship is the only idea that moves him. Against the rabbis he has no complaint to make; with them, he said, he had nothing to do. He thinks that Schwartzberg is extreme and unfair, and that there are good and bad rabbis in New York. He is reserved and undemonstrative, and speaks only in reply. When the rather puzzled visitor asked him if there was anything in which he was interested, he replied, "Yes, in my cyclopedia." The only point at which he betrayed feeling was when he quoted proudly the words of a reviewer of the cyclopedia, who had wondered where Dr. Rosenberg had obtained all his learning. He stated indifferently that the Hebrew language and literature is dead and cannot be revived. "I know," he said, "that Hebrew literature does not pay, but I cannot stop." With no indignation, he remarked that the Jews in New York have no ideals. It was a fact objectively to be deplored, but for which he personally had no emotion, all of that being reserved for his cyclopedia.

These three men are perfect types of the "submerged Hebrew scholar" of the New York Ghetto. Reicherson is the typical religious teacher; Schwartzberg, the enthusiast, who loves the language like a mistress, and Rosenberg, the cool "man of wisdom," who only cares for the perfection of knowledge. Altho there are several others on the East Side who approach the type, they fall more or less short of it. Either they are not really scholars in the old tongue, altho reading and even writing it, or through business or otherwise they have raised themselves above the pathetic point. Thus Dr. Benedict Ben-Zion, one of the poorest of all, being reduced to occasional tutoring, and the sale of a patent medicine for a living, is not specifically a scholar. He writes and reads Hebrew, to be sure, but is also a playwright in the "jargon"; has been a Christian missionary to his own people in Egypt, Constantinople, and Rumania, a doctor for many years, a teacher in several languages, one who has turned his hand to everything, and whose heart and mind are not so purely Hebraic as those of the men I have mentioned. He even is seen, more or less, with Ghetto *literati* who are essentially hostile to what the true Hebrew scholar holds by—a body of Russian Jewish socialists of education, who in their Grand and Canal Street cafés express every night in impassioned language their contempt for whatever is old and historical.

Then, there are J. D. Eisenstein, the youngest and one of the most learned, but perhaps the least "submerged" of them all; Gerson Rosenschweig, a wit, who has collected the epigrams of the Hebrew literature, added many of his own, and written in Hebrew a humorous treatise on America—a very up-to-date Jew, who, like Schwartzberg, tried to run a Hebrew weekly, but when he failed, was not discouraged, and turned to business and politics instead; and Joseph Low Sossnitz, a very learned scholar, of dry and sarcastic tendency, who only recently has risen above the submerged point. Among the latter's most notable published books are a philosophical attack on materialism, a treatise on the sun, and a work on the philosophy of religion.

It is the wrench between the past and the present which has placed these few scholars in their present pathetic condition. Most of them are old, and when they die the "maskil" as a type will have vanished from New York. In the meantime, tho they starve, they must devote themselves to the old language, the old

137

ideas and traditions of culture. Their poet, the austere Dolitzki, famous in Russia at the time of the revival of Hebrew twenty years ago, is the only man in New York who symbolizes in living verse the spirit in which these old men live, the spirit of love for the race as most purely expressed in the Hebrew literature. This disinterested love for the remote, this pathetic passion to keep the dead alive, is what lends to the lives of these "submerged" scholars a nobler quality than what is generally associated with the East Side.

The rabbis, as well as the scholars, of the East Side of New York have their grievances. They, too, are "submerged," like so much in humanity that is at once intelligent, poor, and out-of-date. As a lot, they are old, reverend men, with long gray beards, long black coats and little black caps on their heads. They are mainly very poor, live in the barest of the tenement houses and pursue a calling which no longer involves much honor or standing. In the old country, in Russia—for most of the poor ones are Russian—the rabbi is a great person. He is made rabbi by the state and is rabbi all his life, and the only rabbi in the town, for all the Jews in every city form one congregation, of which there is but one rabbi and one cantor. He is a man always full of learning and piety, and is respected and supported comfortably by the congregation, a tax being laid on meat, salt, and other foodstuffs for his special benefit.

But in New York it is very different. Here there are hundreds of congregations, one in almost every street, for the Jews come from many different cities and towns in the old country, and the New York representatives of every little place in Russia must have their congregation here. Consequently, the congregations are for the most part small, poor and unimportant. Few can pay the rabbi more than $3 or $4 a week, and often, instead of having a regular salary, he is reduced to occasional fees for his services at weddings, births and holy festivals generally. Some very poor congregations get along without a rabbi at all, hiring one for special occasions, but these are congregations which are falling off somewhat from their orthodox strictness.

The result of this state of affairs is a pretty general falling off in the character of the rabbis. In Russia they are learned men— know the Talmud and all the commentaries upon it by heart— and have degrees from the rabbinical colleges, but here they are often without degrees, frequently know comparatively little about the Talmud, and are sometimes actuated by worldly motives. A few Jews coming to New York from some small Russian town will often select for a rabbi the man among them who knows a little more of the Talmud than the others, whether he has ever studied for the calling or not. Then, again, some mere adventurers get into the position—men good for nothing, looking for a position. They clap a high hat on their heads, impose on a poor congregation with their up-to-dateness and become rabbis without learning or piety. These "fake" rabbis—"rabbis for business only"—are often satirized in the Yiddish plays given at the Bowery theatres. On the stage they are ridiculous figures, ape American manners in bad accents, and have a keen eye for gain.

The genuine, pious rabbis in the New York Ghetto feel, consequently, that they have their grievances. They, the accomplished interpreters of the Jewish law, are well-nigh submerged by the frauds that flood the city. But this is not the only sorrow of the "real" rabbi of the Ghetto. The rabbis uptown, the rich rabbis, pay little attention to the sufferings, moral and physical, of their downtown brethren. For the most part the uptown rabbi is of the German, the downtown rabbi of the Russian branch of the Jewish race, and these two divisions of the Hebrews hate one another like poison. Last winter when Zangwill's dramatized *Children of the Ghetto* was produced in New York the organs of the swell uptown German-Jew protested that it was a pity to represent faithfully in art the sordidness as well as the beauty of the poor Russian Ghetto Jew. It seemed particularly baneful that the religious customs of the Jews should be thus detailed upon the stage. The uptown Jew felt a little ashamed that the proletarians of his people should be made the subject of literature. The downtown Jews, the Russian Jews, however, received play and stories with delight, as expressing truthfully their life and character, of which they are not ashamed.

Another cause of irritation between the downtown and uptown rabbis is a difference of religion. The uptown rabbi, representing congregations larger in this country and more American in comfort and tendency, generally is of the "reformed" complexion, a hateful thought to the orthodox downtown rabbi, who is loath to admit that the term rabbi fits these swell German preachers. He maintains that, since the uptown rabbi is, as a rule, not only "reformed" in faith, but in preaching as well, he is in reality no rabbi, for, properly speaking, a rabbi is simply an interpreter of the law, one with whom the Talmudical wisdom rests, and who alone can give it out; not one who exhorts, but who, on application, can untie knotty points of the law. The uptown rabbis they call "preachers," with some disdain.

So that the poor, downtrodden rabbis—those among them who look upon themselves as the only genuine—have many annoyances to bear. Despised and neglected by their rich brethren, without honor or support in their own poor communities, and surrounded by a rabble of unworthy rivals, the "real" interpreter of the "law" in New York is something of an object of pity.

Just who the most genuine downtown rabbis are is, no doubt, a matter of dispute. I will not attempt to determine, but will quote in substance a statement of Rabbi Weiss as to genuine rabbis, which will include a curious section of the history of the Ghetto. He is a jolly old man, and smokes his pipe in a tenement-house room containing 200 books of the Talmud and allied writings.

A genuine rabbi [he said] knows the law, and sits most of the time in his room, ready to impart it. If an old woman comes in with a goose that has been killed, the rabbi can tell her, after she has explained how the animal met its death, whether or not it is *kosher*, whether it may be eaten or not. And on any other point of diet or general moral or physical hygiene the rabbi is ready to explain the law of the Hebrews from the time of Adam until to-day. It is he who settles many of the quarrels of the neighborhood. The poor sweat-shop Jew comes to complain of his "boss," the old woman to tell him her dreams and get his interpretation of them, the young girl to weigh with him questions of amorous eitquette. Our children do not need to go to the Yiddish theatres to learn about "greenhorn" types. They see all sorts of Ghetto Jews in the house of the rabbi, their father.

I myself was the first genuine rabbi on the East Side of New York. I am now sixty-two years old, and came here sixteen years ago— came for pleasure, but my wife followed me, and so I had to stay.

[Here the old rabbi smiled cheerfully.] When I came to New York, I found the Jews here in a very bad way—eating meat that was "thrapho," not allowed, because killed improperly; literally, killed by a brute. The slaughter-houses at that time had no rabbi to see that the meat was properly killed, was *kosher*—all right.

You can imagine my horror. The slaughter-houses had been employing an orthodox Jew, who, however, was not a rabbi, to see that the meat was properly killed, and he had been doing things all wrong, and the chosen people had been living abominably. I immediately explained the proper way of killing meat, and since then I have regulated several slaughter-houses and make my living in that way. I am also rabbi of a congregation, but it is so small that it doesn't pay. The slaughter-houses are more profitable.

These "submerged" rabbis are not always quite fair to one another. Some East Side authorities maintain that the "orthodox Jew" of whom Rabbi Weiss spoke thus contemptuously, was one of the finest rabbis who ever came to New York, one of the most erudite of Talmudic scholars. Many congregations united to call him to America in 1887, so great was his renown in Russia. But when he reached New York the general fate of the intelligent adult immigrant overtook him. Even the "orthodox" in New York looked upon him as a "greenhorn" and deemed his sermons out-of-date. He was inclined, too, to insist upon a stricter observance of the law than suited their lax American ideas. So he, too, famous in Russia, rapidly became one of the "submerged."

One of the most learned, dignified and impressive rabbis of the East Side is Rabbi Vidrovitch. He was a rabbi for forty years in Russia, and for nine years in New York. Like all true rabbis he does not preach, but merely sits in his home and expounds the "law." He employs the Socratic method of instruction, and is very keen in his indirect mode of argument. Keenness, indeed, seems to be the general result of the hair-splitting rabbinical education. The uptown rabbis, "preachers," as the downtown rabbi contemptuously calls them, send many letters to Rabbi Vidrovitch seeking his help in the untying of knotty points of the "law." It was from him that Israel Zangwill, when the *Children*

141

of the Ghetto was produced on the New York stage, obtained a minute description of the orthodox marriage ceremonies. Zangwill caused to be taken several flash-light photographs of the old rabbi, surrounded by his books and dressed in his official garments.

There are many congregations in the New York Ghetto which have no rabbis and many rabbis who have no congregations. Two rabbis who have no congregations are Rabbi Beinush and Rabbi, or rather, Cantor, Weiss. Rabbi Weiss would say of Beinush that he is a man who knows the Talmud, but has no diploma. Rabbi Beinush is an extremely poor rabbi with neither congregation nor slaughter-houses, who sits in his poor room and occasionally sells his wisdom to a fishwife who wants to know if some piece of meat is *kosher* or not. He is down on the rich uptown rabbis, who care nothing for the law, as he puts it, and who leave the poor downtown rabbi to starve.

Cantor Weiss is also without a job. The duty of the cantor is to sing the prayer in the congregation, but Cantor Weiss sings only on holidays, for he is not paid enough, he says, to work regularly, the cantor sharing in this country a fate similar to that of the rabbi. The famous comedian of the Ghetto, Mogolesco, was, as a boy, one of the most noted cantors in Russia. As an actor in the New York Ghetto he makes twenty times as much money as the most accomplished cantor here. Cantor Weiss is very bitter against the uptown cantors: "They shorten the prayer," he said. "They are not orthodox. It is too hot in the synagogue for the comfortable uptown cantors to pray."

Comfortable Philistinism, progress and enlightenment uptown; and poverty, orthodoxy and patriotic and religious sentiment, with a touch of the material also, downtown. Such seems to be the difference between the German and the Russian Jew in this country, and in particular between the German and Russian Jewish rabbi.

Altho Abraham Cahan began his literary career as a Yiddish writer for the Ghetto newspapers his important work has been written and published in English. His work as a Yiddish writer was of an almost exclusively educational character. This at once establishes an important distinction between him and the Yiddish sketch-writers considered in the foregoing section. A still more vital distinction is that arising from the relative quality of his work, which as opposed to that of the Yiddish writers, is more of the order of the story or of the novel than of the sketch. Cahan's work is more developed and more mature as art than that of the other men, who remain essentially sketch-writers. Even in their longer stories what is good is the occasional flash of life, the occasional picture, and this does not imply characters and theme developed sufficiently to put them in the category of the novel. Rather than for the art they reveal they are interesting for the sincere way in which they present a life intimately known. In fact the literary talent of the Ghetto consists almost exclusively in the short sketch. To this general rule Abraham Cahan comes the nearest to forming an exception. Even in his work the sketch element predominates; but in one long story at least something more is successfully achieved; in his short stories there is often much circumstance and development; and he has now finished the first draft of a long novel. His stories have appeared from time to time in the leading English magazines, and there are two volumes with which the discriminating American and English public is familiar, *Yekl* and *The Imported Bridegroom and Other Stories*. As well as his work Cahan's life too is of unusual interest. He had a picturesque career as a socialist and an editor in the Ghetto.

Abraham Cahan was born in Vilna, the capital of Lithuania, Russia, in 1860. He went as a boy to the Jewish "chaider," but took an early and overpowering interest in the Russian language and ideas. He graduated from the *Teacher's Institute* at Vilna, and was appointed government teacher in the town of Velizh, Province of Vitebsk. Here he became interested, altho not active, in the anarchistic doctrines which filled the intellectual atmosphere of the day; and, feeling that his liberty and activity were endangered by a longer sojourn in Russia, he came to America in 1882, when a time of severe poverty and struggle ensued.

From the first he, like most Russian Jews of intelligence, was identified with the socialist movement in the New York Ghetto; he threw himself into it with extraordinary activity and soon became a leader in the quarter. He was an eloquent and impassioned speaker, went twice abroad as the American-Jewish delegate to socialist congresses, and was the most influential man connected with the weekly *Arbeiterzeitung,* of which he became editor in 1893. This paper, as has been explained, for several years carried on an aggressive warfare in the cause of labor and socialism, and attempted also to educate the people to an appreciation of the best realistic Russian writers, such as Tolstoi, Turgenieff and Chekhov. It was under Cahan's editorship of this weekly, and also of the monthly *Zukunft,* a journal of literature and social science, that some of the realistic sketch-writers of the quarter discovered their talent; and for a time both literature and socialism were as vigorous as they were young in the colony.

Literature, however, was at that time to Cahan only the handmaiden of education. His career as an East Side writer was that primarily of the teacher. He wished not merely to educate the ignorant masses of the people in the doctrines of socialism, but to teach them the rudiments of science and literature. For that reason he wrote in the popular "jargon," popularized science, wrote socialistic articles, exhorted generally. Occasionally he published humorous sketches, intended, however, always to point a moral or convey some needed information. In literature, as such, he was not at that time interested as an author. It was only several years later, when he took up his English pen, that he attempted to put into practise the ideas about what constitutes real literature to which he had been trying to educate the Ghetto.

The fierce individualism which in spite of socialistic doctrine is a characteristic of the intellectual element in the Ghetto soon brought about its weakening effects. The inevitable occurred. Quarrels grew among the socialists, the party was split, each faction organized a socialist newspaper, and the movement consequently lost in significance and general popularity. In 1896 Cahan resigned his editorship, and retired disgusted from the work.

From that time on his interest in socialism waned, altho he still ranges himself under that banner; and his other absorbing interest, realistic literature, grew apace, until it now absorbs everything else. As is the case with many imaginative and emotional men he is predominantly of one intellectual passion. When he was an active socialist he wanted to be nothing else. He gave up his law studies, and devoted himself to an unremunerative public work. When the fierce but small personal quarrels began which brought about the present confused condition of socialism in the Ghetto, Cahan's always strong admiration for the Russian writers of genius and their literary school led him to experiment in the English language, which gave a field much larger than the "jargon." Always a reformer, always filled with some idea which he wished to propagate through the length and breadth of the land, Cahan took up the cause of realism in English fiction with the same passion and energy with which he had gone in for socialism. He became a partisan in literature just as he had been a partisan in active life. He admired among Americans W. D. Howells, who seemed to him to write in the proper spirit, but he felt that Americans as a class were hopelessly "romantic," "unreal," and undeveloped in their literary tastes and standards. He set himself to writing stories and books in English which should at least be genuine artistic transcripts from life, and he succeeded admirably in keeping out of his work any obvious doctrinaire element—which points to great artistic self-restraint when one considers how full of his doctrine the man is.

Love of truth, indeed, is the quality which seems to a stranger in the Ghetto the great virtue of that section of the city. Truth, pleasant or unpleasant, is what the best of them desire. It is true that, in the reaction from the usual "affable" literature of the American book-market, these realists rather prefer the unpleasant. That, however, is a sign of energy and youth. A vigorous youthful literature is always more apt to breathe the spirit of tragedy than a literature more mature and less fresh. And after all, the great passion of the intellectual quarter results in the consciously held and warmly felt principle that literature should be a transcript from life. Cahan represents this feeling in its purest aspect; and is therefore highly interesting not only as a man but as a type. This passion for truth is deeply infused into his literary work.

The aspects of the Ghetto's life which would naturally hold the interest of the artistic observer are predominatingly its characteristic features—those qualities of character and conditions of social life which are different from the corresponding ones in the old country. Cahan came to America a mature man with the life of one community already a familiar thing to him. It was inevitable therefore that his literary work in New York should have consisted largely in fiction emphasizing the changed character and habits of the Russian Jew in New York; describing the conditions of immigration and depicting the clash between the old and the new Ghetto and the way the former insensibly changes into the latter. In this respect Cahan presents a great contrast to the simple Libin, who merely tells in a heartfelt passionate way the life of the poor sweat-shop Jew in the city, without consciously taking into account the relative nature of the phenomena. His is absolute work as far as it goes, as straight and true as an arrow, and implies no knowledge of other conditions. Cahan presents an equally striking contrast to the work of men like Gordin and Gorin, the best part of which deals with Russian rather than New York life.

If Cahan's work were merely the transcribing in fiction form of a great number of suggestive and curious "points" about the life of the poor Russian Jew in New York, it would not of course have any great interest to even the cultivated Anglo-Saxon reader, who, tho he might find the stories curious and amusing for a time, would recognize nothing in them sufficiently familiar to be of deep importance to him. If, in other words, the stories had lacked the universal element always present in true literature they would have been of very little value to anyone except the student of queer corners. When however the universal element of art is present, when the special conditions are rendered sympathetic by the touch of common human nature, the result is pleasing in spite of the foreign element; it is even pleasing because of that element; for then the pleasure of easily understanding what is unfamiliar is added to the charm of recognizing the old objects of the heart and the imagination.

Cahan's stories may be divided into two general classes: those presenting primarily the special conditions of the Ghetto to which the story and characters are subordinate; and those in which the special conditions and the story fuse together and mutually help and explain one another. These two—the "information" element and the "human nature" element—struggle for the mastery throughout his work. In the most successful part of the stories the "human nature" element masters, without suppressing, that of special information.

The substance of Cahan's stories, what they have deliberately to tell us about the New York Ghetto, is, considering the limited volume of his work, rich and varied. It includes the description of much that is common to the Jews of Russia and the Jews of New York—the picture of the orthodox Jew, the pious rabbi, the marriage customs, the religious holidays, etc. But the orthodox foreign element is treated more as a background on which are painted in contrasting lights the moral and physical forms resulting from the particular colonial conditions. The falling away of the children in filial respect and in religious faith, the consequent despair of the parents, who are influenced only in superficial ways by their new environment; the alienation of "progressive" husbands from "old-fashioned" wives; the institution of "the boarder," a source of frequent domestic trouble; the tendency of the "new" daughters of Israel to select husbands for themselves in spite of ancient authority and the "Vermittler," and their ambition to marry doctors and lawyers instead of Talmudical scholars; the professional letter-writers through whom ignorant people in the old country and their ignorant relatives here correspond; the falling-off in respect for the Hebrew scholar and the rabbi, the tendency to read in the Astor Library and do other dreadful things implying interest in American life, to eat *treife* food, talk American slang, and hate being called a "greenhorn," *i.e.*, an old-fashioned Jew; how a "Mister" in Russia becomes a "Shister" (shoemaker) in New York, and a "Shister" in Russia becomes a "Mister" in New York; how women lay aside their wigs and men shave their beards and ride in horse-cars on Saturday: all these things and more are told in more or less detail in Cahan's English stories. Anyone who followed the long series of Barge Office sketches which during the last few years Cahan has published anonymously in the *Commercial Advertiser,* would be familiar in a general way with the different types of Jews who come to this country, with the reasons for their immigration and

147

the conditions which confront them when they arrive. Many of these hastily conceived and written newspaper reports have plenty of life—are quick, rather formless, flashes of humor and pathos, and contain a great deal of implicit literature. But the salient quality of this division of Cahan's work is the amount of strange and picturesque information which it conveys.

Many of his more carefully executed stories which have appeared from time to time in the magazines are loaded down with a like quantity of information, and while all of them have marked vitality, many are less intrinsically interesting, from the point of view of human nature, than even the Barge Office sketches. A marked instance of a story in which the information element overpoweringly predominates is "The Daughter of Reb Avrom Leib," published in the *Cosmopolitan Magazine* for May, 1900. The tale opens with a picture of Aaron Zalkin, who is lonely. It is Friday evening, and for the first time since he left his native town he enters a synagogue. Then we have a succession of minutely described customs and objects which are interesting in themselves and convey no end of "local color." We learn that orthodox Jewish women have wigs, we read of the Holy Ark, the golden shield of David, the illuminated *omud,* the reading platform in the centre, the faces of the worshippers as they hum the Song of Songs, and then the cantor and the cantor's daughter. We follow the cantor in his ceremonies and prayers. Zalkin is thrilled by the ceremony and thrilled by the girl. But only a word is given to him before the story goes back to picturing the scene, Reb Avrom Leib's song and the actions of the congregation. In the second division of the story Zalkin goes again the next Friday night to the synagogue, and the result is that he wants to marry the girl. So he sends a "marriage agent" to the cantor, the girl's father. Then he goes to "view the bride," and incidentally we learn that the cantor has two sons who are "American boys," and "will not turn their tongues to a Hebrew word." When the old man finds that Zalkin is a Talmudic scholar he is startled and delighted and wants him for a son-in-law. They try to outquote one another, shouting and gesticulating "in true Talmudic fashion." There is a short scene between the two young people, the wedding-day is deferred till the "Nine Days" are over, for "who would marry

148

while one was mourning the Fall of the Temple?" And it is suggested that Sophie is not quite content. Then there is a scene where Zalkin chants the Prophets, where the betrothal articles, "a mixture of Chaldaic and Hebrew," are read and a plate is thrown on the floor to make a severance of the ceremony "as unlikely as would be the reunion of the broken plate." Then there are more quotations from the cantor, a detailed picture of the services of the Day of Atonement, of the Rejoicing of the Law, blessing the Dedication Lights, the Days of Awe, and the Rejoicing of the Law again. The old man's character is made very vivid, and the dramatic situation—that of a Jewish girl who, after the death of her father, marries in compliance with his desire—is picturesquely handled. But the theme is very slight. Most of the detail is devoted to making a picture, not of the changing emotions in the characters and the development of the human story, but of the religious customs of the Jews. The emphasis is put on information rather than on the theme, and consequently the story does not hold the interest strongly.

Many of Cahan's other short stories suffer because of the learned intention of the author. We derive a great deal of information and we generally get the "picture," but it often requires an effort to keep the attention fixed on what is unfamiliar and at the same time so apart from the substance of the story that it is merely subordinate detail.

In these very stories, however, there is much that is vigorous and fresh in the treatment and characterization; and a vein of lyric poetry is frequent, as in the delightful *Ghetto Wedding*, the story of how a poor young Jewish couple spend their last cent on an elaborate wedding-feast, expecting to be repaid by the presents, and thus enabled to furnish their apartment. The gifts don't turn up, only a few guests are present, and the young people, after the ceremony, go home with nothing but their enthusiastic love. The naïveté and simplicity of the lovers, the implicit sympathy with them, and a kind of gentle satire, make this little story a gem for the poet.

The Imported Bridegroom is a remarkable character sketch and contains several very strong and interesting descriptions. Asriel Stroon is the central figure and lives before the mind of the

149

reader. He is an old Jew who has made a business success in New York, and retired, when he has a religious awakening and at the same time a great longing for his old Russian home Pravly. He goes back to Pravly on a visit, and the description of his sensations the day he returns to his home is one of the best examples of the essential vitality of Cahan's work. This long story contains also a most amusing scene where Asriel outbids a famous rich man of the town for a section in the synagogue and triumphs over him, too, in the question of a son-in-law. There is in Pravly a "prodigy" of holiness and Talmudic learning, Shaya, whom Reb Lippe wants for his daughter, but Asriel wants him too, and being enormously rich, carries him off in triumph to his daughter in America. But Flora at first spurns him. He is a "greenhorn," a scholar, not a smart American doctor such as she has dreamed of. Soon, however, Shaya, who is a great student, learns English and mathematics, and promises Flora to become a doctor. The first thing he knows he is a freethinker and an American, and Flora now loves him. They keep the terrible secret from the old man, but he ultimately sees Shaya going into the Astor Library and eating food in a *treife* restaurant. His resentment is pathetic and intense, but the children marry, and the old man goes to Jerusalem with his faithful servant.

The book, however, in which there is a perfect adaptation of "atmosphere" and information to the dramatic story is *Yekl.* In this strong, fresh work, full of buoyant life, the Ghetto characters and environment form an integral part.

Yekl indeed ought to be well known to the English reading public. It is a book written and conceived in the English language, is essentially idiomatic and consequently presents no linguistic difficulties. It gives a great deal of information about what seems to me by far the most interesting section of foreign New York. But what ought to count more than anything else is that it is a genuine piece of literature; picturing characters that live in art, in an environment that is made real, and by means of a story that is vital and significant and that never flags in interest. In its quality of freshness and buoyancy it recalls the work of Turgenieff. None of Cahan's later work, tho most of it has vital elements, stands in the same class with this fundamentally sweet

150

piece of literature. It takes a worthy place with the best Russian fiction, with that school of writers who make life actual by the sincere handling of detail in which the simple everyday emotions of unspoiled human nature are portrayed. The English classic novel, greatly superior in the rounded and contemplative view of life, has yet nothing since Fielding comparable to Russian fiction in vivid presentation of the details of life. This whole school of literature can, I believe, be compared in quality more fittingly with Elizabethan drama than anything which has intervened in English literature; not of course with those maturer dramas in which there is a great philosophical treatment of human life, but in the lyric freshness and imaginative vitality which were common to the whole lot of Elizabethan writers.

Yekl is alive from beginning to end. The virtuosity in description which in Cahan's work sometimes takes the place of literature, is here quite subordinate. Yekl is a sweat-shop Jew in New York who has left a wife and child in Russia in order to make a little home for them and himself in the new world. In the early part of the book he is becoming an "American" Jew, making a little money and taking a great fancy to the smart Jewish girl who wears a "rakish" hat, no wig, talks "United States," and has a profound contempt for the benighted pious "greenhorns" who have just arrived. A sweat-shop girl named Mamie moves his fancy deeply, so that when the faithful wife Gitl and the little boy Yossele arrive at the Barge Office there is evidently trouble at hand. At that place Yekl meets them in a vividly told scene—ill-concealed disquiet on his part and naïve alarm at the situation on hers. Gitl's wig and her subdued, old-fashioned demeanor tell terribly on Yekl's nerves, and she is shocked by everything that happens to her in America. Their domestic unhappiness develops through a number of characteristic and simple incidents until it results in a divorce. But by that time Gitl is becoming "American" and it is obvious that she is to be taken care of by a young man in the quarter more appreciative than Yekl. The latter finds himself bound to Mamie, the pert "American" girl, and as the book closes is in a fair way to regret the necessity of giving up his newly acquired freedom. This simple, strong theme is treated consistently in a vital presentative way. The idea is developed by

151

natural and constant incident, psychological or physical, rather than by talk. Every detail of the book grows naturally out of the situation.

"Unpleasant" is a word which many an American would give to *Yekl* on account of its subject. Strong compensating qualities are necessary to induce a publisher or editor to print anything which they think is in subject disagreeable to the big body of American readers, most of whom are women. Without attempting to criticise the "voice of the people," it may be pointed out that there are at least two ways in which a book may be "unpleasant." It may be so in the formal theme, the characters, the result—things may come out unhappily, vice triumphant, and the section of life portrayed may be a sordid one. This is the kind of unpleasantness which publishers particularly object to; and in this sense *Yekl* may fairly be called "unpleasant." Turgenieff's *Torrents of Spring* is also in this sense "unpleasant," for it tells how a young man's sincere and poetic first love is turned to failure and misery by the illegitimate temporary attraction of a fascinating woman of the world. But Turgenieff's novel is nevertheless full of buoyant vitality, full of freshness and charm, of youth and grace, full of life-giving qualities; because of it we all may live more abundantly. The same may be said of many another book. When there is sweetness, strength and early vigor in a book the reader is refreshed notwithstanding the theme. And it is noticeable that youth is not afraid of "subjects."

Another way in which a book may be "unpleasant" is in the quality of deadness. Many books with pleasant and moral themes and endings are unpoetic and unpleasantly mature. Even a book great in subject, with much philosophy in it, may show a lack of sensitiveness to the vital qualities, to the effects of spring, to the joy in mere physical life, which are so marked and so genuinely invigorating in the best Russian fiction. The extreme of this kind of unpleasantness is shown in the case of some modern Frenchmen and Italians; not primarily in the theme, but in the lack of poetry and vigor, of hope; in a sodden maturity, often indeed combined with great qualities of intellect and workmanship, but dead to the little things of life, dead to the feeling of spring in the blood, to naïve readiness for experience. An American who is the antithesis of this kind of thing is Walt Whitman. His quality put into prose is what we have in the best Russian novels. In the latter acceptation of the word unpleasant, too, it cannot be applied to *Yekl;* for *Yekl* is youthful and vital. There is buoyant spring in the lines and robust joy in truth whatever it may be.

Apropos of Cahan's love of truth, and that word "unpleasant," a discussion which took place a few years ago on the appearance of Zangwill's play *Children of the Ghetto,* is illuminative. That poetic drama represented the life of the poor Ghetto Jew with sympathy and truth; but for that very reason it was severely criticised by some uptown Israelites. Many of these, no doubt, had religious objections to a display on the stage of those customs and observances of their race which touched upon the "holy law." But some of the rich German Jews, practically identified with American life, and desiring for practical and social purposes to make little of their racial distinction, deprecated literature which portrayed the life of those Jews who still have distinctively national traits and customs. Then, too, there is a tendency among the well-to-do American Jews to look down upon their Ghetto brethren, to regard the old customs as benighted and to treat them with a certain contempt; altho they spend a great deal of charitable money in the quarter. Feeling a little ashamed of the poor Russian East Side Jew, they object to a serious literary portrayal of him. They want no attention called to what they deem the less attractive aspects of their race. An uptown Jewish lady, on the appearance in a newspaper of a story about East Side Jewish life, wrote a protesting letter to the editor. She told the writer of the sketch, when he was sent to see her, that she could not see why he didn't write about uptown Jews instead of sordid East Side Jews. The scribe replied that he wrote of the Ghetto Jew because he found him interesting, while he couldn't see anything attractive or picturesque about the comfortable Israelite uptown.

Abraham Cahan's stories have been subjected to criticism inspired by the same spirit. Feeling the charm of his people he has attempted to picture them as they are, in shadow and light; and has consequently been accused of betraying his race to the Gentiles.

The attitude of the East Side Jews towards writers like Zangwill and Cahan is in refreshing contrast. The Yiddish newspapers were enthusiastic about *Children of the Ghetto,* in which they felt the Jews were truthfully and therefore sympathetically portrayed. In the literary sketches and plays now produced in considerable numbers in the "jargon," a great pride of race is manifest. The writers have not lost their self-respect, still abound in their own sense and are consequently vitally interesting. They are full of ideals and enthusiasm and do not object to what is "unpleasant" so strenuously as do their uptown brethren.

Morris Rosenfeld, poet and former tailor, strikes in his personality and writings the weary minor. Full of tears are the man and his song. Zunser, Dolitzki, and Wald, altho in their verse runs the eternal melancholy of poetry and of the Jews, have yet physical buoyancy and a robust spirit. But Rosenfeld, small, dark, and fragile in body, with fine eyes and drooping eyelashes, and a plaintive, childlike voice, is weary and sick—a simple poet, a sensitive child, a bearer of burdens, an East Side tailor. Zunser and Dolitzki have shown themselves able to cope with their hard conditions, but the sad little Rosenfeld, unpractical and incapable in all but his songs, has had the hardest time of all. His life has been typical of that of many a delicate poet—a life of privation, of struggle borne by weak shoulders, and a spirit and temperament not fitted to meet the world.

Much younger than Zunser or Dolitzki, Morris Rosenfeld was born thirty-eight years ago in a small village in the province of Subalk, in Russian Poland, at the end of the last Polish revolution. The very night he was born the world began to oppress him, for insurgents threw rocks through the window. His grandfather was rich, but his father lost the money in business, and Morris received very little education—only the Talmud and a little German, which he got at a school in Warsaw. He married when he was sixteen, "because my father told me to," as the poet expressed it. He ran away from Poland to avoid being pressed into the army. "I would like to serve my country," he said, "if there had been any freedom for the Jew." Then he went to Holland and learned the trade of diamond-cutting; then to London, where he took up tailoring.

Hearing that the tailors had won a strike in America, he came to New York, thinking he would need to work here only ten hours a day. "But what I heard," he said, "was a lie. I found the sweat-shops in New York just as bad as as they were in London."

In those places he worked for many years, worked away his health and strength, but at the same time composed many a sweetly sad song. "I worked in the sweat-shop in the daytime," he said to me, "and at night I worked at my poems. I could not help writing them. My heart was full of bitterness. If my poems are sad and plaintive, it is because I expressed my own feelings, and because my surroundings were sad."

Next to Zunser, Rosenfeld is the most popular of the four Jewish poets. Zunser is most popular in Russia, Rosenfeld in this country. Both write in the universal Yiddish or "jargon," both are simple and spontaneous, musical and untutored. But, unlike Zunser, Rosenfeld is a thorough representative, one might say victim, of the modern spirit. Zunser sings to an older and more buoyant Jewish world, to the Russian Hebrew village and the country at large. Rosenfeld in weary accents sings to the maimed spirit of the Jewish slums. It is a fresh, naïve note, the pathetic cry of the bright spirit crushed in the poisonous air of the Ghetto. The first song that Rosenfeld printed in English is this:

> I lift mine eyes against the sky,
> The clouds are weeping, so am I;
> I lift mine eyes again on high,
> The sun is smiling, so am I.
> Why do I smile? Why do I weep?
> I do not know; it lies too deep.

> I hear the winds of autumn sigh,
> They break my heart, they make me cry;
> I hear the birds of lovely spring,
> My hopes revive, I help them sing.
> Why do I sing? Why do I cry?
> It lies so deep, I know not why.

*   *   *   *   *   *   *

In the three Yiddish theatres on the Bowery is expressed the world of the Ghetto—that New York City of Russian Jews, large, complex, with a full life and civilization. In the midst of the frivolous Bowery, devoted to tinsel variety shows, "dive" music-halls, fake museums, trivial amusement booths of all sorts, cheap lodging-houses, ten-cent shops and Irish-American tough saloons, the theatres of the chosen people alone present the serious as well as the trivial interests of an entire community. Into these three buildings crowd the Jews of all the Ghetto classes—the sweat-shop woman with her baby, the day-laborer, the small Hester Street shopkeeper, the Russian-Jewish anarchist and socialist, the Ghetto rabbi and scholar, the poet, the journalist. The poor and ignorant are in the great majority, but the learned, the intellectual and the progressive are also represented, and here, as elsewhere, exert a more than numerically proportionate influence on the character of the theatrical productions, which, nevertheless, remain essentially popular. The socialists and the literati create the demand that forces into the mass of vaudeville, light opera, historical and melodramatic plays a more serious art element, a simple transcript from life or the theatric presentation of a Ghetto problem. But this more serious element is so saturated with the simple manners, humor and pathos of the life of the poor Jew, that it is seldom above the heartfelt understanding of the crowd.

The audiences vary in character from night to night rather more than in an uptown theatre. On the evenings of the first four week-days the theatre is let to a guild or club, many hundred of which exist among the working people of the East Side. Many are labor organizations representing the different trades, many are purely social, and others are in the nature of secret societies. Some of these clubs are formed on the basis of a common home in Russia. The people, for instance, who came from Vilna, a city in the old country, have organized a Vilna Club in the Ghetto. Then, too, the anarchists have a society; there are many socialistic orders; the newspapers of the Ghetto have their constituency, which sometimes hires the theatre. Two or three hundred dollars is paid to the theatre by the guild, which then sells the tickets among the faithful for a good price. Every member of the society is forced to buy, whether he wants to see the play or not, and the money made over and above the expenses of hiring the theatre is for the benefit of the guild. These performances are therefore called "benefits." The widespread existence of such a custom is a striking indication of the growing sense of corporate interests among the laboring classes of the Jewish East Side. It is an expression of the socialistic spirit which is marked everywhere in the Ghetto.

On Friday, Saturday and Sunday nights the theatre is not let, for these are the Jewish holidays, and the house is always completely sold out, altho prices range from twenty-five cents to a dollar. Friday night is, properly speaking, the gala occasion of the week. That is the legitimate Jewish holiday, the night before the Sabbath. Orthodox Jews, as well as others, may then amuse themselves. Saturday, altho the day of worship, is also of holiday character in the Ghetto. This is due to the Christian influences, to which the Jews are more and more sensitive. Through economic necessity Jewish workingmen are compelled to work on Saturday, and, like other workingmen, look upon Saturday night as a holiday, in spite of the frown of the orthodox. Into Sunday, too, they extend their freedom, and so in the Ghetto there are now three popularly recognized nights on which to go with all the world to the theatre.

On those nights the theatre presents a peculiarly picturesque sight. Poor workingmen and women with their babies of all ages fill the theatre. Great enthusiasm is manifested, sincere laughter and tears accompany the sincere acting on the stage. Pedlars of soda-water, candy, of fantastic gewgaws of many kinds, mix freely with the audience between the acts. Conversation during the play is received with strenuous hisses, but the falling of the curtain is the signal for groups of friends to get together and gossip about the play or the affairs of the week. Introductions are not necessary, and the Yiddish community can then be seen and approached with great freedom. On the stage curtain are advertisements of the wares of Hester Street or portraits of the "star" actors. On the programmes and circulars distributed in the audience are sometimes amusing announcements of coming attractions or lyric praise of the "stars." Poetry is not infrequent, an example of which, literally translated, is:

157

Labor, ye stars, as ye will,
Ye cannot equal the artist;
In the garden of art ye shall not flourish;
Ye can never achieve his fame.
Can you play *Hamlet* like him?
The *Wild King*, or the *Huguenots?*
Are you gifted with feeling
So much as to imitate him like a shadow?
Your fame rests on the pen;
On the show-cards your flight is high;
But on the stage every one can see
How your greatness turns to ashes,
Thomashevsky! Artist great!
No praise is good enough for you;
Every one remains your ardent friend.
Of all the stars you remain the king.
You seek no tricks, no false quibbles;
One sees Truth itself playing.
Your appearance is godly to us;
Every movement is full of grace;
Pleasing is your every gesture;
Sugar-sweet your every turn;
You remain the King of the Stage;
Everything falls to your feet.

On the playboards outside the theatre, containing usually the portrait of a star, are also lyric and enthusiastic announcements. Thus, on the return of the great Adler, who had been ill, it was announced on the boards that "the splendid eagle has spread his wings again."

The Yiddish actors, as may be inferred from the verses quoted, take themselves with peculiar seriousness, justified by the enthusiasm, almost worship, with which they are regarded by the people. Many a poor Jew, man or girl, who makes no more than $10 a week in the sweat-shop, will spend $5 of it on the theatre, which is practically the only amusement of the Ghetto Jew. He has not the loafing and sporting instincts of the poor Christian, and spends his money for the theatre rather than for drink. It is not only to see the play that the poor Jew goes to the theatre. It is to see his friends and the actors. With these latter he, and more frequently she, try in every way to make acquaintance, but commonly are compelled to adore at a distance. They love the songs that are heard on the stage, and for these the demand is so great that a certain bookshop on the East Side makes a speciality of publishing them.

The actor responds to this popular enthusiasm with sovereign contempt. He struts about in the cafés on Canal and Grand Streets, conscious of his greatness. He refers to the crowd as "Moses" with superior condescension or humorous vituperation. Like thieves, the actors have a jargon of their own, which is esoteric and jealously guarded. Their pride gave rise a year or two ago to an amusing strike at the People's Theatre. The actors of the three Yiddish companies in New York are normally paid on the share rather than the salary system. In the case of the company now at the People's Theatre, this system proved very profitable. The star actors, Jacob Adler and Boris Thomashevsky, and their wives, who are actresses—Mrs. Adler being the heavy realistic tragedienne and Mrs. Thomashevsky the star soubrette—have probably received on an average during that time as much as $125 a week for each couple. But they, with Mr. Edelstein, the business man, are lessees of the theatre, run the risk and pay the expenses, which are not small. The rent of the theatre is $20,000 a year, and the weekly expenses, besides, amount to about $1,100. The subordinate actors, who risk nothing, since they do not share the expenses, have made amounts during this favorable period ranging from $14 a week on the average for the poorest actors to $75 for those just beneath the "stars." But, in spite of what is exceedingly good pay in the Bowery, the actors of this theatre formed a union, and struck for wages instead of shares. This, however, was only an incidental feature. The real cause was that the management of the theatre, with the energetic Thomashevsky at the head, insisted that the actors should be prompt at rehearsals, and if they were not, indulged in unseemly epithets. The actors' pride was aroused, and the union was formed to insure their ease and dignity and to protect them from harsh words. The management imported actors from Chicago. Several of the actors here stood by their employers, notably Miss Weinblatt, a popular young ingénue, who, on account of her great memory is called the "Yiddish Encyclopedia," and Miss Gudinski, an actress of commanding presence. Miss Weinblatt forced her father, once an actor, now a farmer, into the service of the management. But the actors easily triumphed. Misses Gudinski and Weinblatt were forced to join the union, Mr. Weinblatt returned to his farm, the "scabs" were packed off to Philadelphia, and the wages system introduced. A delegation was sent to Philadelphia to throw cabbages at the new actors, who appeared in the Yiddish performances in that city. The triumphant actors now receive on the average probably $10 to $15 a week less than under the old system. Mr. Conrad, who began the disaffection, receives a salary of $29 a week, fully $10 less than he received for months before the strike. But the dignity of the Yiddish actor is now placed beyond assault. As one of them recently said: "We shall no longer be spat upon nor called 'dog.' "

The Yiddish actor is so supreme that until recently a regular system of hazing playwrights was in vogue. Joseph Latteiner and Professor M. Horowitz were long recognized as the only legitimate Ghetto playwrights. When a new writer came to the theatre with a manuscript, various were the pranks the actors would play. They would induce him to try, one after another, all the costumes in the house, in order to help him conceive the characters; or they would make him spout the play from the middle of the stage, they themselves retiring to the gallery to "see how it sounded." In the midst of his exertions they would slip away, and he would find himself shouting to the empty boards. Or, in the midst of a mock rehearsal, some actor would shout, "He is coming, the great Professor Horowitz, and he will eat you"; and they would rush from the theatre with the panic-stricken playwright following close at their heels.

The supremacy of the Yiddish actor has, however, its humorous limitations. The orthodox Jews who go to the theatre on Friday night, the beginning of Sabbath, are commonly somewhat ashamed of themselves and try to quiet their consciences by a vociferous condemnation of the actions on the stage. The actor, who through the exigencies of his rôle, is compelled to appear on Friday night with a cigar in his mouth, is frequently greeted with hisses and strenuous cries of "Shame, shame, smoke on the Sabbath!" from the proletarian hypocrites in the gallery.

The plays at these theatres vary in a general way with the varying audiences of which I have spoken above. The thinking socialists naturally select a less violent play than the comparatively illogical anarchists. Societies of relatively conservative Jews desire a historical play in which the religious Hebrew in relation to the persecuting Christian is put in pathetic and melodramatic situations. There are a very large number of "culture" pieces produced, which, roughly speaking, are plays in which the difference between the Jew of one generation and the next is dramatically portrayed. The pathos or tragedy involved in differences of faith and "point of view" between the old rabbi and his more enlightened children is expressed in many historical plays of the general character of *Uriel Acosta*, tho in less lasting form. Such plays, however, are called "historical plunder" by that very up-to-date element of the intellectual Ghetto which is dominated by the Russian spirit of realism. It is the demand of these fierce realists that of late years has produced a supply of theatrical productions attempting to present a faithful picture of the actual conditions of life. Permeating all these kinds of plays is the amusement instinct pure and simple. For the benefit of the crowd of ignorant people grotesque humor, popular songs, vaudeville tricks, are inserted everywhere.

Of these plays the realistic are of the most value, for they often give the actual Ghetto life with surprising strength and fidelity. The past three years have been their great seasons, and have developed a large crop of new playwrights, mainly journalists who write miscellaneous articles for the East Side newspapers. Jacob Gordin, of whom we shall have frequent occasion to speak, has been writing plays for several years, and was the first realistic playwright; he remains the strongest and most prominent in this kind of play. Professor Horowitz, who is now the lessee of the Windsor Theatre, situated on the Bowery, between Grand and Canal Streets, represents, along with Joseph Latteiner, the conservative and traditional aspects of the stage. He is an interesting

161

man, fifty-six years of age, and has been connected with the
Yiddish stage practically since its origin. His father was a teacher
in a Hebrew school, and he himself is a man of uncommon
learning. He has made a great study of the stage, has written one
hundred and sixty-seven plays, and claims to be an authority on
dramaturgie. Latteiner is equally productive, but few of their
plays are anything more than Yiddish adaptations of old operas
and melodramas in other languages. Long runs are impossible on
the Yiddish stage and consequently the playwrights produce
many plays and are not very scrupulous in their methods. The
absence of dramatic criticism and the ignorance of the audience
enable them to "crib" with impunity. As one of the actors said,
Latteiner and Horowitz and their class took their first plays from
some foreign source and since then have been repeating themselves. The actor said that when he is cast in a Latteiner play he
does not need to learn his part. He needs only to understand the
general situation; the character and the words he already knows
from having appeared in many other Latteiner plays.

The professor, nevertheless, naturally regards himself and Latteiner as the "real" Yiddish playwrights. For many years after the
first bands of actors reached the New York Ghetto these two men
held undisputed sway. Latteiner leaned to "romantic," Horowitz
to "culture," plays, and both used material which was mainly
historical. The professor regards that as the bright period of the
Ghetto stage. Since then there has been, in his opinion, a
decadence which began with the translation of the classics into
Yiddish. *Hamlet, Othello, King Lear*, and plays of Schiller, were
put upon the stage and are still being performed. Sometimes they
are almost literally translated, sometimes adapted until they are
realistic representations of Jewish life. Gordin's *Yiddish King
Lear*, for instance, represents Shakespeare's idea only in the most
general way, and weaves about it a sordid story of Jewish character and life. Of *Hamlet* there are two versions, one adapted, in
which Shakespeare's idea is reduced to a ludicrous shadow, the
interest lying entirely in the presentation of Jewish customs.

The first act of the Yiddish version represents the wedding
feast of Hamlet's mother and uncle. In the Yiddish play the uncle
is a rabbi in a small village in Russia. He did not poison Hamlet's

father but broke the latter's heart by wooing and winning his queen. Hamlet is off somewhere getting educated as a rabbi. While he is gone his father dies. Six weeks afterwards the son returns in the midst of the wedding feast, and turns the feast into a funeral. Scenes of rant follow between mother and son, Ophelia and Hamlet, interspersed with jokes and sneers at the sect of rabbis who think they communicate with the angels. The wicked rabbi conspires against Hamlet, trying to make him out a nihilist. The plot is discovered and the wicked rabbi is sent to Siberia. The last act is the graveyard scene. It is snowing violently. The grave is near a huge windmill. Ophelia is brought in on the bier. Hamlet mourns by her side and is married, according to the Jewish custom, to the dead woman. Then he dies of a broken heart. The other version is almost a literal translation. To these translations of the classics, Professor Horowitz objects on the ground that the ignorant Yiddish public cannot understand them, because what learning they have is limited to distinctively Yiddish subjects and traditions.

Another important step in what the professor calls the degeneration of the stage was the introduction a few years ago of the American "pistol" play—meaning the fierce melodrama which has been for so long a characteristic of the English plays produced on the Bowery.

But what has contributed more than anything else to what the good man calls the present deplorable condition of the theatre was the advent of realism. "It was then," said the professor one day with calm indignation, "that the genuine Yiddish play was persecuted. Young writers came from Russia and swamped the Ghetto with scurrilous attacks on me and Latteiner. No number of the newspaper appeared that did not contain a scathing criticism. They did not object to the actors, who in reality were very bad, but it was the play they aimed at. These writers knew nothing about *dramaturgie,* but their heads were filled with senseless realism. Anything historical and distinctively Yiddish they thought bad. For a long time Latteiner and I were able to keep their realistic plays off the boards, but for the last few years there has been an open field for everybody. The result is that horrors under the mask of realism have been put upon the stage. This

year is the worst of all—characters butchered on the stage, the
coarsest language, the most revolting situations, without ideas,
with no real material. It cannot last, however. Latteiner and I
continue with our real Yiddish plays, and we shall yet regain
entire possession of the field."

At least this much may fairly be conceded to Professor Horowitz—that the realistic writers in what is in reality an excellent
attempt often go to excess, and are often unskilful as far as stage
construction is concerned. In the reaction from plays with
"pleasant" endings, they tend to prefer equally unreal "unpleasant" endings, "onion" plays, as the opponents of the realists
call them. They, however, have written a number of plays which
are distinctively of the New York Ghetto, and which attempt an
unsentimental presentation of truth. Professor Horowitz's plays,
on the contrary, are largely based upon the sentimental repre-
sentation of inexact Jewish history. They herald the glory and
wrongs of the Hebrew people, and are badly constructed melodramas of conventional character. Another class of plays written
by Professor Horowitz, and which have occasionally great but
temporary prosperity, are what he calls *Zeitstucke*. Some American newspaper sensation is rapidly dramatized and put hot on
the boards, such as *Marie Barberi, Dr. Buchanan* and *Dr. Har-
ris*.

The three theatres—the People's, the Windsor and the Thalia,
which is on the Bowery opposite the Windsor—are in a general
way very similar in the character of the plays produced, in the
standard of acting and in the character of the audience. There
are, however, some minor differences. The People's is the "swellest" and probably the least characteristic of the three. It panders
to the "uptown" element of the Ghetto, to the downtown trades-
man who is beginning to climb a little. The baleful influence in
art of the *nouveaux riches* has at this house its Ghetto expression.
There is a tendency there to imitate the showy qualities of the
Broadway theatres—melodrama, farce, scenery, etc. No babies
are admitted, and the house is exceedingly clean in comparison
with the theatres farther down the Bowery. Three years ago this
company were at the Windsor Theatre, and made so much money
that they hired the People's, that old home of Irish-American

melodrama, and this atmosphere seems slightly to have affected the Yiddish productions. Magnificent performances quite out of the line of the best Ghetto drama have been attempted, notably Yiddish dramatizations of successful uptown productions. Hauptman's *Versunkene Glocke, Sappho, Quo Vadis,* and other popular Broadway plays in flimsy adaptations were tried with little success, as the Yiddish audiences hardly felt themselves at home in these unfamiliar scenes and settings.

The best trained of the three companies is at present that of the Thalia Theatre. Here many excellent realistic plays are given. Of late years, the great playwright of the colony, Jacob Gordin, has written mainly for this theatre. There, too, is the best of the younger actresses, Mrs. Bertha Kalisch. She is the prettiest woman on the Ghetto stage and was at one time the leading lady of the Imperial Theatre at Bucharest. She takes the leading woman parts in plays like *Fedora, Magda* and *The Jewish Zaza.* The principal actor at this theatre is David Kessler, who is one of the best of the Ghetto actors in realistic parts, and one of the worst when cast, as he often is, as the romantic lover. The actor of most prominence among the younger men is Mr. Moshkovitch, who hopes to be a "star" and one of the management. When the union was formed he was in a quandary. Should he join or should he not? He feared it might be a bad precedent, which the actors would use against him when he became a star. And yet he did not want to get them down on him. So before he joined he entered solemn protests at all the cafés on Canal Street. The strike, he maintained, was unnecessary. The actors were well paid and well treated. Discipline should be maintained. But he would join because of his universal sympathy with actors and with the poor— as a matter of sentiment merely, against his better judgment.

The company at the Windsor is the weakest, so far as acting is concerned, of the three. Very few "realistic" plays are given there, for Professor Horowitz is the lessee, and he prefers the historical Jewish opera and "culture" plays. Besides, the company is not strong enough to undertake successfully many new productions, altho it includes some good actors. Here Mrs. Prager vies as a prima donna with Mrs. Karb of the People's and Mrs. Kalisch of the Thalia. Professor Horowitz thinks she is far

165

better than the other two. As he puts it, there are two and a half prima donnas in the Ghetto—at the Windsor Theatre there is a complete one, leaving one and a half between the People's and the Thalia. Jacob Adler of the People's, the professor thinks, is no actor, only a remarkable caricaturist. As Adler is the most noteworthy representative of the realistic actors of the Ghetto, the professor's opinion shows what the traditional Yiddish playwright thinks of realism. The strong realistic playwright, Jacob Gordin, the professor admits, has a "biting" dialogue, and "unconsciously writes good cultural plays which he calls realistic, but his realistic plays, properly speaking, are bad caricatures of life."

The managers and actors of the three theatres criticise one another indeed with charming directness, and they all have their followers in the Ghetto and their special cafés on Grand or Canal Streets, where their particular prejudices are sympathetically expressed. The actors and lessees of the People's are proud of their fine theatre, proud that no babies are brought there. There is a great dispute between the supporters of this theatre and those of the Thalia as to which is the stronger company and which produces the most realistic plays. The manager of the Thalia maintains that the People's is sensational, and that his theatre alone represents true realism; while the supporter of the People's points scornfully to the large number of operas produced at the Thalia. They both unite in condemning the Windsor, Professor Horowitz's theatre, as producing no new plays and as hopelessly behind the times, "full of historical plunder." An episode in *The Ragpicker of Paris*, played at the Windsor when the present People's company were there, amusingly illustrates the jealousy which exists between the companies. An old beggar is picking over a heap of moth-eaten, coverless books, some of which he keeps and some rejects. He comes across two versions of a play, *The Two Vagrants*, one of which was used at the Thalia and the other at the Windsor. The version used at the Windsor receives the beggar's commendation, and the other is thrown in a contemptuous manner into a dust-heap.

LOUIS MARSHALL

Louis Marshall, from whose *Public Papers*, edited by Charles Reznikoff, the following selection is taken, was so eminent a legal figure in his generation that serious consideration was given to him, we are told, as the first Jew to be appointed to the bench of the Supreme Court of the United States before that honor went to Louis D. Brandeis.

Louis Marshall: Champion of Liberty
(*Edited by Charles Reznikoff*)

Jacob Joseph, chief rabbi of the Russian Jewish Orthodox congregations in New York City, died July 28, 1902. Only a handful of police, in spite of notice that the funeral procession would be numerous, was assigned to it to keep order. It was estimated, afterwards, that 20,000 were in the procession. They crowded the street, from curb to curb, for the length of four blocks. As the procession passed the factory of R. Hoe and Company, manufacturers of printing-presses, it was jeered at by apprentices and workingmen and met with screws, bolts, and nuts from the upper windows.

A complaint by a committee was received politely in the office of the factory but without results. Angry mourners burst into the place. They were swept out by the use of a fire-hose, and other fire-hose from the factory drenched those outside. By this time, stones and other missiles were thrown at the building from the street. However, the riot was soon over. Then the police reserves arrived and began clubbing mourners and spectators.

Mayor Seth Low appointed a committee of five—including Louis Marshall—to investigate the incident and its wider implications of police inefficiency and brutality—particularly towards the Jews of the East Side. (The report of the committee is to be found in the *American Hebrew* for September 19, 1902, pp. 497-499.)

Writing to R. E. Carey on January 23, 1905, Marshall said:

. . . You are somewhat in error, in saying that Mayor Low took no

Selection from *Louis Marshall: Champion of Liberty*, edited by Charles Reznikoff. Published by the Jewish Publication Society, Philadelphia, 1957.

notice of the attack on the funeral procession of Rabbi Joseph. He appointed a commission to investigate it, of which the late William H. Baldwin, Jr., Messrs. Edward B. Whitney, Nathan Bijur, Thomas Mulry and I were members. There was a very full report rendered, a number of policemen were disciplined, the blame was placed where it belonged, the captain who was guilty of dereliction of duty resigned, an inspector was put on trial, and the effect has been most salutary, the Jewish people being now protected by the police against similar outrages, where before, their complaints were unnoticed. Moreover, they now receive better treatment in the police courts, whereas, prior to this episode, they were treated with brutality by everybody connected with many of those courts, from the magistrates down.

December 29, 1902

To the Editors, Jewish Gazette

In reply to yours of the 28th inst., asking me to state my opinion regarding the unsuccessful termination of the proceedings instituted against the accused public officers, I wish to say that while I am somewhat disappointed at the fact that there have been no convictions, I nevertheless believe that the effect of the agitation and investigation which followed the occurrences at Rabbi Joseph's funeral has been most wholesome and that there is no occasion to fear a repetition of the offences which so greatly moved the entire community last summer.

It is always difficult to convict a public officer either before a jury or before the head of a department. Witnesses are apt to forget; to become indifferent; to evade the performance of their public obligations. Those in charge of the prosecution are frequently handicapped and do not receive the moral support which is always essential to success. On the other hand, those who are proceeded against are always able to enlist the assistance and support of their friends; to gather about them earnest helpers and to command witnesses. Their forces are united and are actuated by the motive of self-preservation, while those of the prosecution are scattered.

This experience is not confined to prosecutions of the character which we now have under consideration. Even in cases where there have been convictions for crimes which have attracted much public attention and in which new trials have been granted by the appellate courts on the ground of technical errors committed at the trial, it seems to be practically impossible to secure a conviction on a retrial.

But even though there have been no convictions in the present instance it does not follow that the Jewish community should be discouraged, or even feel that its rights have been disregarded. On the contrary, it was demonstrated to the satisfaction of the entire world that the infamous charges that had been made, that the Jews were the aggressors, were utterly without foundation. Furthermore, the public authorities recognized it to be their duty to thoroughly investigate the affair and to place the blame where it belonged. Such investigation took place and the responsibility was fixed after a thorough and impartial hearing.

The press of the entire country with remarkable unanimity and without regard to political or other affiliations condemned those who were responsible for the wanton attack upon the funeral procession, and the police who either from carelessness, indifference or brutality rendered the occurrences of that occasion possible.

In this country public opinion is the greatest power for good, and there can be no doubt that the public opinion of this country will not tolerate a repetition of such an offence as that of last summer. As a consequence the rights of the Jews will be better safe-guarded than they could be by an army of soldiers, and the police authorities will recognize their obligations and the necessity of treating the residents of the East Side with humanity and the consideration which they deserve.

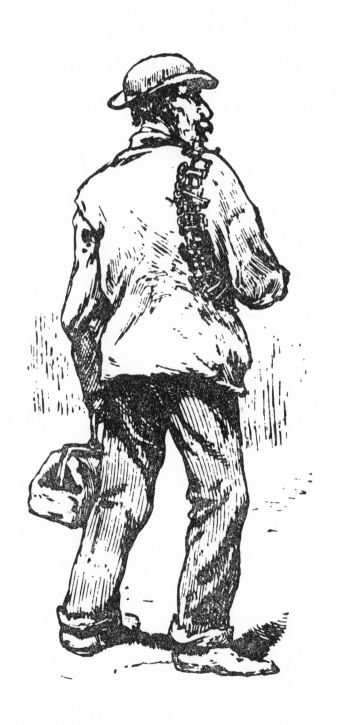

MAURICE HINDUS

Maurice Hindus was born in
a small village in Russia in 1891. In his autobiography, he describes his father as a "koolak" who was something of a contra-
diction to the conventional conception of that term, as it was
defined after the Bolshevik Revolution: "At one time he possessed ten horses, twenty cows, many calves, geese and hens, and
he was the only farmer in the village who threshed his grain not
with flails but with a horse-drawn threshing machine built of
heavy timbers—the sole mark of the machine age in the community. Banned because of his Jewish faith from owning land
except for a house and a garden, he rented a large acreage from
the noted Count Radzivill. Had he been an energetic and competent businessman with an eye for financial gain, he could have
whipped a fortune out of Radzivill's land. As it was, the count's
acres proved a stupendous liability and in the end ruined him and
his family."

After the death of his improvident father (who married twice
and had seventeen children), Maurice came with his mother and
brothers and sisters to the United States in 1905. While the rest
of the family, like most other immigrants of the period, stayed on
in New York City where they had landed, his own ill-health and
dissatisfaction with what he saw of the ghetto life (which he
describes in the chapters selected for inclusion in this anthology)
caused him to leave for upstate New York, where he went to work
on a farm. He managed to put himself through Colgate College,
where he was elected to Phi Beta Kappa. After doing graduate
work at Harvard University, from which he took a master's de-

gree, he published his first book at the age of twenty-nine, *The Russian Peasant and the Revolution.* It was received very favorably; one of the professors who reviewed it thought its analysis so sound that it would still be readable in a hundred years.

After successfully completing a journalistic assignment from *Century Magazine* to cover the story of the Tolstoyan colony of Doukhobor peasants who had settled in Canada, he made his first trip back to Russia in the early 1920's. Out of his observations grew the book *Broken Earth,* introduced to American readers by John Dewey. Hindus is the author of twenty books, most of them accounts of his travels in Russia but also including two novels and an autobiography. Two of his books deal with Czechoslovakia where he reported the Sudeten crisis with Hitlerite Germany in 1938 and from which he received in grateful recognition for his services the Czechoslovak State Prize for Literature (this award came from democratic Czechoslovakia; the Communists, after their takeover, were to accuse him of spying on behalf of the Zionists and the United States). One of his books, *In Search of a Future,* deals with his travels in the countries of the Middle East including Israel.

Seventeen of his books concern Russia in one way or another. The most widely known is probably *Humanity Uprooted.* which Justice Holmes mentions, in his correspondence with Harold Laski, having read at the suggestion of his Supreme Court colleague Brandeis. The book also led to his meeting with the novelist F. Scott Fitzgerald, at the latter's request, in Baltimore in 1930. Hardly less well-known and popular in their time were his books *Red Bread, The Great Offensive* and *Mother Russia.* His latest works are *House Without a Roof,* which received the Overseas Press Association award for the best foreign reporting in 1962, and his recent book *The Kremlin's Human Dilemma.* He has received an Honorary Doctorate in Literature from his alma mater, Colgate University.

Maurice Hindus is one of those who has taken to heart Tolstoy's warning to historians in *War and Peace* that, in studying society, they must make their observations focus not upon the nominal leaders of a country but upon its common people. He says: "Through all the years, since 1923, that I have been intimately observing the Soviet Union, my chief concern has been not with economics, politics, doctrine, but with people, more notably with the peasantry." The single-minded insistence with which he has taken this point of view has led to some criticism among his peers in the study of Russia, even when these have recognized and paid tribute to the quality, brilliance, and profundity of the work he has done. But this pertinacity is also probably responsible for the fact that he has been on occasion the most reliable prophet of coming events, as when he dared to predict in the title of a book, published soon after June 22, 1941, and the subject of some derision by reviewers like Clifton Fadiman for its lack of hardheaded realism, *Hitler Cannot Conquer Russia*, or when much later on he predicted the fall of Khrushchev when the latter was at the height of his power on the basis of the failure of his agricultural policy. In an Appendix to one of his books, *Crisis in the Kremlin*, he produced a painstaking piece of historical research establishing beyond cavil Russian responsibility in starting the Korean conflict in 1950. In the opinion of many qualified observers, his books have been probably the most illuminating and instructive analyses of the effects of the Russian Revolution over a period of fifty years that have been produced in the United States.

Green Worlds

Often I wonder whether it was our village that discovered America or whether it was America that discovered our village! Either proposition can be argued with facility and vehemence, though neither is susceptible of mathematical proof. I have the feeling that the feverish energies of America, reaching out first for our bristles and our flax, had at least as much to do with it as the boisterous curiosity of our villagers.

At any rate, I had been in this country, or rather in New York, less than a week when the evidence in support of all the legends I had heard of America from beggars, gypsies, lumbermen, peddlers, merchants and other impassioned gatherers of news reached overwhelming proportions. Fat meat, for example. I am sure that Ivan the Fool, who in disgust, because of his ineligibility for admission, denounced every good word on America as a deliberate and malicious fraud, would have gasped with delight at a mere glance at the meat that I had for my first meal. Of course it was fat. The sight of the roast sputtering with hot grease stirred me to ecstasy. In the old home I had never had enough meat. No matter how heartily I had eaten I could always dispose of another helping of meat, especially if it was fatty. I readily ate the sausage of our neighbors, without Mother knowing it, of course, because of the little balls of fat that shone out of it like stars in a murky sky. Now fat meat was mine for the asking, and, what was more, I learned that it was cheaper than lean meat, a strange subversion of good taste, I thought. I hurried with my first help-

Selections from Maurice Hindus' *Green Worlds*, published by Doubleday, New York, 1938.

176

ing so as to be sure I would be in time for another before it was all consumed.

Yet the thrill did not last long. Soon I not only wearied of fat meat, but I lost all appetite for it—it died as completely as our bonfires in the woods when a shower splashed down. I got so that on being asked whether I cared for the fat portion of a roast I shook my head in fullhearted refusal. In the stern climate of the old village, where the mud alone sharpened the appetite, and where little of it was to be had, and where the amount of other fats was limited, fat meat was an aspiration and a boon. But in New York, with its mild weather and its abundance of fats in other foods, it became an ordeal. I should not have minded had there been a law banning its sale or even its use.

All that I had heard of sugar was true. If at home only lumbermen and merchants and landlords might allow themselves the luxury of sweetening their tea by dropping sugar into the glass, two and three or more lumps, here even I might do it without invoking a reprimand or even a look of disapproval from Mother or anyone else in the family. In fact here it was impossible to economize on sugar by nibbling at it as we did at home. There the sugar had a stern geologic quality. Many were the mouthfuls of hot tea that passed over it before it eroded into complete dissolution. If I held the piece that I hacked off with my teeth under the tongue, I might drink half a glass of tea before the taste of sweetness in my mouth was washed away. Here, whether I held the piece under or over the tongue, on mere contact with a mouthful of hot tea its cohesiveness collapsed as readily as the lump of half-dried mud with which, out of spite or revenge, I used to smite the back or the face of a playmate. Here it took less sugar to sweeten the tea in the glass than in the mouth. That was the kind of sugar America had, but there was lots of it, and it was cheap, and its use in the accepted form meant no special extravagance.

True also were the stories of white bread. At first I could not eat enough of it—sweet rolls, plain rolls, with cinnamon and poppy seeds, without cinnamon and poppy seeds; I ate them during meals and between meals. In walking the streets and seeing displays in bakeries or on pushcarts I often yielded to the

177

temptation of indulging the appetite for them. Yet soon enough, as in the case of fat meat, I tired of white bread. Often I wished I could drop in on Boris the Cattle, as poor a man as there was in the village, ask him to cut me a slab of black bread, retire to a corner beside his huge brick oven and make a meal of it with a cucumber or with nothing more than garlic rubbed on the crusted part. Baked with grated potato instead of with yeast, which the village had not yet discovered, and never fresh except on the day it came out of the oven, its very solidity and coarseness gave it a tang and a relish which the puffy and overrefined American bread never had. I was amazed at my sudden hunger for the black bread of the old days.

Magnificently true were the stories of handkerchiefs and shoes. Here even I had to have a handkerchief, and not only on the Sabbath and on holidays but on weekdays. The sleeve of the blouse or the bare hand might do well enough in the old village, but not in the streets or anywhere else in New York. A woman just could not stoop down and reach for the bottom of her dress, as she might do in the old village, every time she wanted to blow her nose. Nor did girls need to wait for marriage to flaunt a handkerchief before neighbors and make them aware of the good fortune that had come to them. A handkerchief was neither luxury nor adornment, nor badge of superiority, and one needed to be neither landlord nor merchant to be supplied with one at all times and for all emergencies.

And of course nobody walked barefooted nor in *lapti*—not even children, not in the street, anyway; nor did anybody clump about in thick-leathered knee-high boots; and, whatever the shoes that a man wore, he never bothered to soil his hands, the floor, his clothes, by applying grease to them and then wait for hours or overnight for it to soak into the leather and dry before again stepping into them. He got "a shine" while sitting in a comfortable chair, and when he descended to the sidewalk and looked at his shoes, his heart thumped with joy, for they gleamed like mirrors, and no one in the old home, neither the landlord nor the lumberman nor any of the officials in swanky uniforms, ever could make their boots glisten so brilliantly. Most true was the story of cigarette paper, too true. Nobody used wrapping paper, copybook paper, newspaper, for the rolling of cigarettes and, what was more, hardly anybody made his own, anyway. A man bought his cigarettes ready-made and in pretty boxes. Back home neither the landlord's sons nor daughters, when they went riding horseback and smoked, displayed such cigarettes or such pretty boxes.

Shockingly false, of course, was the story of the colors of American pants. True, people did not make them of white home-spun or factory-woven linen, nor did they in their choice of fabrics compete for color with buttercups, cornflowers, lilacs, as did our village landlords and their children in the trousers they sported when they went riding horseback. The dark gray of the home-woven woolen cloth, were it not so hot and heavy, would have won complete approval in America. Indeed, instead of talking so much about bright-colored pants, our folk in the old village might better have learned something of the glories of American underwear. Here was something to stir anyone's fancy. The mere contact of the garment with the body gave a man a feeling of gallantry. He could spread his legs, twist his limbs, crawl, climb, jump over beds, chairs, stand on his head, roll on the floor, and yet when he dashed before a mirror to look at himself the suit clung to him as trim and tight as the skin of an apple. Their ignorance of underwear would have made the story all the more exciting to the folk in the old home.

It was just as well, of course, that nobody had ever mumbled a word about bananas. Not only Ivan the Fool, but Blind Sergey as well, would have twisted his face in revulsion. He might have deemed the fruit excellent forage for the Evil One, or perhaps discovered in it the surest means of exorcising his presence from the community. Until the time that he had acquired a taste for it he would have thought it no more fit for human consumption than a green thistle. Subsequently he might regret the initial revulsion, but then Blind Sergey was no novice at subsequent regrets.

Our villagers might have heard a few words of other American achievements—of the little shiny bars of chocolate, for example, that beckoned to the pedestrian from endless pushcarts on the streets. Sold at a penny—that is, at two kopecks apiece—the poorest boy in the old village could have purchased one or several, at least on the eve of a holiday, for the girl whose hand he hoped to win. The gift would have evoked endless exclamations of gratitude and would have aided the suit more brilliantly than freshly picked cucumbers, or lumps of sugar. Had Anna been around, I should have loaded her hands with the shiny little bars. No doubt she would have treasured them so highly that she would have eaten them with black bread, perhaps only on Sundays and for dessert.

Our people might likewise have heard a few words of the soda fountains that gleamed majestically out of the open stalls and in the candy shops and spouted the palate-pricking carbonated water into a large glass at a price no higher than that of a bar of chocolate on the pushcarts, or at twice that amount when seasoned with a lavish portion of rich and fragrant syrup. And why hadn't anyone ever mentioned the decorative and juice-soaked tomato? Not even the German landlord had yet begun to cultivate it, though it would have made a fit companion to the cucumber, because it could be eaten with bread and potato, made into soup and pickle, served with meat and herring, used as an appetizer after a gulp of vodka, munched as a delicacy in between meals and a special boon for the numerous fast days when neither milk nor meat foods nor eggs were permitted. It might even vie with the cucumber in its appeal to girls at a dance or any other gathering.

Had any of my old neighbors followed me around on my rambles in the streets and peered as I did into the shop windows, they would have been as excited as I was and as bewildered by the arrays of foods in cans, in boxes, in jars, in bottles, in packages, in bags, and by the ornate displays of footwear, clothes, haberdashery, hardware, musical instruments and a multitude of other commodities, of the names and uses of which they might have been as ignorant as I was. They would have been as mystified too by the variety and multitude of tastes and appetites that man had acquired in this thunderous America, so many indeed that they would have wondered how people found the time to indulge the one or the other or even to think of them.

Perhaps, though, it was well that they had heard no more than they had. Out of sheer envy or incredulity they might have swung

to the support of Ivan the Fool, who had proclaimed the existence of America an invention and a fraud. Besides, the more
meager the information of those who came over, the more overwhelming would be their joy in the discovery of this fantastic
material abundance. Only then, in the light of the opulence of
America, could they envisage the real destitution of the old village, of the whole world out of which they had come. What
destitution! No socks, no handkerchiefs, no underwear, seldom
enough soap, generations behind the New World, and with no
visible hope of putting itself in a position to reach out for the
knowledge, the energy, the ambition to transform itself to anything similar. How could it, steeped as it was in "the deep and
horrible mud," as my mother would say, and all that it implied in
daily living? It was hard enough to pull cows and horses and
wagons and sometimes our own feet out of that black muck. To
lift the whole scheme of living out of it would have required a
power that was nowhere in sight, a power that could blow the
mud off the face of the earth.

After I had been in New York a few weeks I went to work as
errand boy in a shop. One of my duties was to buy lunches for
the girls who worked there—that is, for those who did not bring
theirs from home. Until I came, this chore had been performed
by an Italian girl named Lina. Bright-eyed, with a mass of dark
hair and wearing a loose and flaming red blouse and a dark skirt,
she was one of the most cheerful girls I had ever known. She
worked with her mother as a button sewer, and to my inexperi-
enced eyes she was as dexterous with needle and thread as her
mother, though her mother was so steeped in her work that she
seldom looked up from the garment in her hands, while Lina,
nimbly plying the needle and thread with her fingers, often
enough swept the room with her brilliant and merry eyes. The
moment anyone caught her glance she broke into a titter. Only
about two years older than myself, her whole life seemed an
endless flow of mirth.

The first day I was in the shop Lina taught me how to go about
getting lunches for the girls. Paper and pencil in hand, she made
the rounds of the girls and wrote down their orders. I envied her

181

the ease and fluency with which she wrote English. Now and
then, as she wrote down a word, she would say something to me,
only to be answered by a look of bafflement, because I understood hardly a word of what she was saying. That gave her an
excuse for an extra giggle. After she had written down all the
orders she went with me to the lunch counter a few doors away
from the shop. On our way she again tried to draw me into
conversation, but I only shook my head and we both laughed.
When the orders were filled we went back to the shop and, by
means of nods, winks, gestures, Lina enabled me properly to
distribute the packages.

The next day I went around taking the orders without Lina's
help. I wrote down the words as I heard them and in Russian. At
the lunch shop I read them off from my piece of paper, and the
fat man at the counter opened a barrage of talk which was as
meaningless to me as Lina's and infinitely more annoying.
Snatching the paper from my hand, he scrutinized it closely,
scowled, shrugged his shoulders and, after more incomprehensi-
ble talk, proceeded to do up the lunches anyway. I was glad Lina
was not along while he was attempting to puzzle out my writing
and to question me as to its contents. She would have screamed
with laughter, and this time it might have been more than embar-
rassing. Still I had the orders filled, and that was a triumph, perhaps a miracle. On my return to the shop I distributed them as
best I could. When the girls opened their packages they turned to
each other with surprise and dismay and proceeded to exchange
sandwiches, pies, cakes. Laughter, scowls, cries of protest, and
Lina in a dither of excitement and, either out of politeness or in
deference to her mother's admonition, heroically suppressing her
mirth. I felt better when her mother called me over to her work
table, gave me a piece of cake and mumbled in sympathy,
"Goota boy, goota boy." Nothing my own mother could have
said in that moment of confusion and pain would have been more
heartening.

The next day Lina went about with me taking the orders and
writing them down on paper. When I came back she helped me to
distribute them to the proper girls. Hearing her repeat the orders
and watching her write them down enabled me to pick up a

substantial vocabulary. In less than a week I could go about and take orders by myself and write them down in English and only rarely get them so badly mixed that the girl who ordered a frank-furter without mustard received a corned-beef sandwich with mustard. Always, of course, Lina with her dancing eyes and her ineffaceable smile was beside me to rectify errors.

Meanwhile, having invested the first week's earnings in a Russian-English dictionary and in a Russian-English study book, I compelled myself every day to commit to memory at least twenty new words. It was fun to come to the shop and to try out my freshly acquired vocabulary on Lina. Patient and amiable, though utterly unable to control her laughter, she took pains to correct my errors, particularly in pronunciation. Her mother knew only a few words of English and smiled with approval on her and on me and often nodded and muttered, "Goota boy, goota boy."

Once I was asked to come in and work on Sunday morning. On my arrival at the shop I found Lina and her mother also there. On finishing work at noon I heard them engage in a spirited dialogue in Italian. I knew it concerned me, because Lina's eyes and smile betrayed her. Then Lina informed me that her mother wanted me to come to their house for lunch. They lived on Mulberry Street, she said, and it would not be much out of my way home, and I didn't have to stay long if I didn't have the time.

Gladly I accepted the invitation and walked with Lina and her mother to Mulberry Street, which was about ten blocks from the shop. After climbing three flights of stairs in an old gas-lighted tenement house, with dark hallways, much darker than in the newer tenement in which I lived, we came to a rear apartment. Lina pounded on the door, and as we entered we were greeted by an explosion of joy which made me forget the dingy and gas-smelling hallways. I had thought that, what with the three boarders who lived with us, our four-room apartment was the very epitome of American overcrowding. Yet here was an Italian household with only three rooms and so many children that I could hardly count them. They seemed to tumble out of chairs, couches, out of the very walls. Nor had I ever known a more noisy or more hilarious family. The adults were only slightly less explosive in their merriment than were the children. The father, a short wiry man with massive shoulders, brilliant eyes, and a face that was a perpetual mask of smiles, greeted me with a prolonged and firm handshake and with a flow of Italian words which I didn't understand and which Lina, with the unsolicited help of her numerous brothers and sisters, hastened to translate for me. Though he had been in this country ten years he had learned only a few more words of English than his wife, but that in no way curbed his exuberant articulateness or his overflowing hospitality. Drawing me to a seat at the table, he passed candy and pastry and poured a glass of wine and bombarded me with questions. His curiosity was as boundless as his cheer. He might have been a peasant in my own old village for all the reserve he showed in his eagerness to learn everything about our family. He was particularly pleased when I told him that my mother had given birth to eleven children, and even more hilarious when I told him that my father had had six more by his first wife. Not everything Lina translated was clear to me. Many of her words and expressions I failed to understand. But words were not as important as gestures, facial expressions, exclamations and, above all, the continuous and explosive roars of laughter. I never had known people who laughed with the energy and enthusiasm of these Italians. They seemed to be born to joy and laughter. I do not remember whether Lina had informed me how many children there were in her family, but I never can forget the thunderous outburst of mirth when her father asked her to tell me that he expected several more. Even the mother joined in the uproar that followed the announcement. Nor did the good man fail to convey to me his hope that when I grew up and got married I should be at least as fecund as my father. When I left and reached the street, I seemed to be billowed along by endless waves of laughter. I wished that people in my part of the city had been as explosively jovial as were Lina and her family.

Shortly afterwards "slack" had set in. Though it was a new word to me, it did not take me long to learn its harrowing meaning. Girl after girl was laid off. Expressmen ceased coming up with cases and rolls of cloth. Fewer and fewer messenger boys called with packages. Finally all the "operators" were told not to come any more. The engine was at a standstill, and so were the machines, and the quiet was at first deafening. Lina and her mother were still needed to sew buttons on the heaps of remaining garments. I too was needed to sweep the floor, fold the garments, pack them into boxes and carry them to the express office. With Lina and her mother around, the shop still had glamor. But soon there were no more garments on which to sew buttons, and Lina and her mother were laid off until the "new season," which might begin in two months and might not start in less than four.

Deserted by my best friends, the shop had lost all brightness and all appeal. It had assumed an air of dismal foreboding. The silent engines and the silent machines were dumb reminders of former struggle and hope. The boss, a huge, phlegmatic man with a bald head and staring eyes, never showed up until midday. He stayed long enough to read his mail, send me down for a corned-beef sandwich and coffee for his lunch and have a few words with the foreman. Only the foreman and I came as usual at an early hour in the morning. A little man with a pinched face and a squeaky voice, the foreman fawned on the boss in the manner of a man who has lost all vestige of self-respect. No muzhik in the old village ever had abased himself so deliberately in the presence of a landlord or a uniformed official as he did before the boss. In mortal dread of losing his job and the wherewithal to support his wife and four children, he resorted to one form of servility after another so as to keep in the good graces of the man on whom the job depended. I wished Lina were around so that I could tell her in my broken English how much I loathed the pathetic little man. But she was gone now. I missed her dancing eyes and her irrepressible laughter, and I missed no less her mother's kindly face and the still more kindly whisper of "Goota boy, goota boy." I felt lonely and forsaken. Soon I too was needed no longer and was dismissed.

Not yet fifteen years of age, I felt deeply the meaning of unemployment in a city. I had been earning only three dollars a week, a small enough sum, but an important item to Mother in

185

her weekly budget. Only by pooling our earnings together, and with her in charge of the housekeeping, could we have the meat and the butter and the other foods that we ate, and of which I had eloquently boasted in letters to former schoolmates in Russia. Mother was urging me to find another job. I tried hard enough. I walked from shop to shop, store to store, one druggist's establishment to another, but no one needed an errand boy whose English was as deficient as mine. I couldn't help wondering what would have happened to me, even if I were grown up, had I been all alone in New York.

In the old village our garden, our few strips of land, our cow, our hens were a guarantee against absolute destitution. Besides, there always was a neighbor who would lend us, or any other family in need, a sack of rye or potatoes until the next harvest was gathered. Even Boris the Cattle or Trofim the Hawk would gladly lend a loaf of bread to a person or a family in want. Poor and backward as we all were, we never starved. In our worst days we never went to bed without the assurance of soup, potatoes and bread for breakfast the next morning. In our simple and primitive economy, unemployment did not matter. Indeed, we hardly knew the meaning of the word. It certainly was no calamity. In winter men loafed most of the time because there was little work for them on the farm. Nor were they overeager to make work for themselves. But they did not suffer from lack of bread, not even in years of a bad harvest. Here, in the moneyed economy of the modern city, his job was all a man had to lean on for his bread. What should I have done without a job? It was well enough to talk of the munificent sums a man could earn in America, all in dollars, and of the multitude of things he could buy at low prices in shops and from pushcarts. But if he lost his job and couldn't find another, no matter how assiduously he searched, what would he do? I dreaded the thought of ever finding myself in such a predicament. True, I was living with a family, but even so, in the moneyed economy of New York and with the low wages my brothers and sisters were receiving, every nickel counted, and every one of us had to earn his own living. The glamor of the American dollar, of which I had heard so much in the old village, vanished, had indeed turned into an evil omen. No, I should never want to be a shopworker, like my older brother and all my sisters. The devil with work in any shop, except as a temporary respite. If only because of the guarantee against destitution which it afforded, I should someday go back to the land. There man never could be as tragically helpless as in the city, with the job in a shop as a sole way of earning a living.

Meanwhile I needed New York, to learn the language and to find my bearings in this stirring new world in which I was to spend the rest of my life.

Every evening I spent hours with my Russian-English dictionary and my Russian-English study book. As soon as I added a few new words to my vocabulary, I hastened to try them on the native-born boys I had met, usually with no end of amusement to them and with no little grief to myself.

Then I entered night school. Nearly all the students were adults, some in their middle age. Working people nearly all of them, after a day's labor in the shop school obviously was too much of a tax on their depleted energies.

In consequence many of them dozed off during the lessons, and then—much to the dismay of the teacher, who to retain his job sought to hold the class together with gymnastic exercises and all manner of promises—one by one they stopped coming. When only a handful of us remained, we were merged with another class. That did not improve our diligence. Students continued to doze off during the lessons and, when called upon to recite or to write a sentence on the blackboard, they wakened with a start, blinked in confusion at the teacher and at the class and remained silent.

I wondered why young boys like myself had to be put in the same classes with grownups, who worked much harder than we did and therefore had less energy and less eagerness for study. I could learn more by poring over my books at home and playing around with the boys I had met on the block or on the roof of our house than in night school, and so I too quit going to classes.

Then I discovered East Broadway. I know of no street in the world which at that time teemed so tempestuously with movements, ideals, ideologies as did this broad and humble thoroughfare in the heart of New York's East Side. Here were Anarchists, Social Revolutionaries, Social Democrats, Social Populists, Zionists, Zangwillites, Assimilationists, Internationalists, Single Taxers, Republicans, Democrats, each group with its own gods, dead and alive, its own demons too, dead and alive, its own headquarters, its own press, its own lectures and debates and its own impassioned resolve to save something or somebody, the working peoples of America, the working peoples of the world, the Russian muzhiks, the Russian proletariat, all the Russian people, the Jews of America, the Jews of the world, the American farmer, the American proletariat, all the American people, all the immigrant peoples. I never had realized that there were so many different ways of achieving salvation or that there were so many people, indeed masses of them, passionately engrossed in bringing it to somebody except to themselves. And lurking in quiet places, in basements, on stoops of houses was another set of crusaders, well-dressed, well-groomed, soft-spoken, always affable and smiling, and they were seeking to save everybody, but especially the immigrant Jews, for Jesus!

It all sounded new and exciting. Earnestly I began to listen to these gospels of hope and deliverance, and the more I listened the more excited and confused I was. I was confronted by a Babel of intellectual tongues, all equally impassioned, equally logical, equally confident of triumph, and equally horrified at the thought of the triumph of the opposition. I was soaking up ideology, all manner of ideology, by the bucketful, and I began to ask myself a multitude of questions which had never before entered my mind. Life had begun to expand. I was becoming aware of ideas and forces outside of myself, of the street on which I lived, of the shop in which I worked, of whose existence and of whose power for good and evil I never had known.

Yet in my boyish naïveté I wondered why these learned folk, who were bursting with ideas, enthusiasm and a spirit of self-sacrifice that often wrung the heart, were so hopelessly divided among themselves. Why did the Anarchists hate the Socialists so vitriolically, and the Socialists the Zionists, and the Nationalists the Internationalists, and the Social Revolutionaries the Social Democrats, and the Single Taxers the Republicans and the Democrats? Love for the ideal fused with a scorching hatred for the opponent. If the crisis in the world was so overwhelming that all mankind, including all of East Broadway, was threatened with collapse and devastation, why didn't these leaders and spokesmen of the new worlds of promise for once sink their differences and pool their wisdom and their energies and hold mankind from the imminent plunge into chaos and ruin? Young as I was, the idea of consecrating oneself to a cause appealed to me. There was excitement and grandeur in a crusade for salvation. The question that tormented me was—which cause to espouse? I shifted from one to another, but none was so foolproof that an older person in a debate with me couldn't demolish, one by one, every tenet that I sought to defend. I gave up in despair. If the prophets of the various causes and their disciples were not wise or strong enough so to fortify their ideological positions that opponents couldn't demolish them, who was I to uphold the beliefs and the aspirations of any of them? I decided that I was neither clever enough nor old and impassioned enough to be a crusader for any abstract ideal.

To this day I wonder why it is that, in a time of crisis, instead of uniting and jointly attacking the common enemy, intellectuals and radicals the world over, unlike reactionaries, persist in fighting and annihilating each other. Witness the bloody internecine feuds in the Christian Revolution, the French Revolution, the Russian Revolution, and even in the budding Spanish Revolution.

It was no use seeking an answer to my perplexing questions. There just was not any. I therefore ceased going to meetings, lectures, debates, and I could no longer be dragged to the cafés where the "gods" gathered and continued their hot feuds to the impassioned delight of their adoring followers.

One evening, in walking along Madison Street, I passed a small, brightly lighted building on the outside of which was an announcement of a lecture on Herbert Spencer by a man named Edward King. The name of Herbert Spencer was new to me, and so was that of the lecturer. I decided to go in. If the man was a good lecturer it would help my English. I slid into a seat in the rear and was surprised at the smallness of the room and of the audience. It was more like a class than a public lecture. The students were all adults and included several women. Not one of the men was in knee pants like myself, which made me a little anxious lest I might be thought an intruder and asked to leave. But no one seemed to be aware of my presence. On a small platform beside a stand piled with books, some of them open, stood a short stocky man with a rolling abdomen and a lofty forehead. He wore glasses, and his eyes were overhung by brows as massive and gray as his mustache. He spoke with a fluency and a fervor that held his audience entranced. So many were the learned words he used that I understood only a small part of what he was saying. Yet I too found myself immersed in the lecture. The warmth of the man, the melodiousness of his voice, the magnificence of his diction stirred me. Sweat shone on his brow, and he frequently wiped it with a handkerchief. On and on he spoke, earnestly, thoughtfully, and neither he nor his audience showed the least fatigue. The thrill of hearing him was all the greater because of my identification of words that I had learned from the dictionary and my study book, but that I had never used and never had heard anyone else use.

When the lecture was finished, the audience gathered around the lecturer and plied him with questions, and the answers constituted another lecture, or rather a series of lectures, for they dealt with a multitude of subjects, some of which had no connection with Herbert Spencer. From their accents alone I could tell that these people were immigrants and, like the lecturer himself but unlike the idealists and the crusaders that I had heard, they were infinitely more concerned with knowledge than with salvation. At any rate, here were no heated arguments and vituperative denunciations of "the enemy," whose scheme of salvation was supposed to plunge all mankind into darkness and woe. They were shopworkers and small businessmen with an uncommon amount of intellectual curiosity.

A little self-conscious, not only because a good part of the conversation was beyond my comprehension but because I was wearing knee pants, I stayed on and listened to the discussion. When the crowd had thinned, the lecturer noticed me—a fresh face—and, reaching out his hand, he greeted me with a hearty handshake and a word of welcome. Then I knew that, so far as he was concerned, my knee pants did not matter. I asked if he had any objection to my coming regularly to his series of lectures on philosophy, and he said no. He asked me a few questions about myself, and I told him that my most pressing task at the moment was to find a job and to master the English language. Forgetting philosophy, he proceeded to offer advice on how best to learn English. Instead of merely memorizing words out of a dictionary and a study book, he suggested that I start reading a book, preferably a novel, because it might be easier to understand and more interesting to follow. Words that I did not know I was to write down on a sheet of paper, and after I had finished reading a page I was to look them up in the dictionary, write out their definitions and memorize them. Then I was to reread the page, and if I understood every word I was to go in the same way with the next page and the next until I finished the book. "But be sure," he warned me, "that you get an interesting book. If you come here next week I'll bring you a book."

Of course I came next week earlier than anybody else, and when he saw me he said, "I have a book for you," and he gave me a secondhand copy of George Eliot's *Adam Bede*. I followed his advice, and to my immense joy my knowledge of the language grew rapidly.

Subsequently I learned something of the history of this singularly learned and lovable man. A Scotsman with a passion for philosophy and an outstanding exponent of positivism, he had settled many years earlier on the East Side and had educated several generations of immigrants. Some of his former pupils and followers, on attaining literary and professional eminence, had raised a modest fund with which to enable him to continue educating fresh groups. He lived in a small apartment on the lower East Side, and his place was a museum of secondhand books. He spent days wandering around old bookshops and buying books that appealed to him even though he knew he should never find the time to read them. They cluttered his rooms and hallways, and when a pupil called he loved to point to them and to talk endlessly of the joy he had in collecting them. His whole life centered in his books, his lectures, his pupils.

I found another job as errand boy in a garment shop, and now my time was divided between work, study, play with the boys on the block, and the weekly lectures of Edward King. I was busy, but I was not happy. I was growing continually aware of an irrepressible conflict between myself and the world about me. If the things that New York displayed to the physical eye, the wonders of the machine age, thrilled, the things that New York was, the New York in which I lived, saddened and dismayed. True enough, I had come from a primitive village where after a rain we were sunk in mud. But our mud did not smell except of dampness. It might give a man heartache but no headache. Yet in the street on which I lived and in the neighboring streets the piles of garbage reeked to heaven and did give me headaches. Why was there so much garbage in the streets? Day and night the piles kept thundering out of stoops and windows. No sooner were the streets cleaned than fresh heaps like foul sores on a diseased body dotted the pavements. Nor were there fields near by and a landlord's forest, as in the old village, to which I might escape.

Of course there was the East River. I discovered it a few days after my arrival. The waterfront was only a few blocks away from the tenement in which I lived, and I often went there for a walk. It was more refreshing to walk there than in any other part of the neighborhood. Yet to me it was no river, not what I had come to regard as a river. Blind Sergey would have yelled his head off that no water nymph would ever want to make her home there. The ferries, tugs, barges and other craft and the smoke that came out of them, which dulled the very shimmer of the waters, would frighten her into flight. Deep enough to swallow many rivers like the one in the old home, it had neither the smell nor the melody of the latter nor its transcendent intimacy and mysteriousness. It might wash away the dirt and sweat of the city, but of the murk which hung over its waters it could not cleanse itself. The very grass on its banks in our neighborhood was entombed in steel and timber. Only after dark, with a breeze blowing off its surface and with the twinkle of the multicolored lights from docks, boats, buildings, did it assume an extraordinary wizardry, and it was more cheering to watch it in the evening than by daylight.

Then I discovered a park with plots of grass and trees, though nothing so luxuriant as the meadows and the birch forests in the old village. Yet every patch of green was stuck with a sign, "Keep Off the Grass." I boiled with indignation. What was a park for if people couldn't sit or lie on the grass in open sunlight or in the shade of a tree? Hot with protest, I jumped over the fence and stretched out full length and gazed at the river ahead. I had lain there only a few minutes when I heard a gruff voice shouting at me. Turning, I saw a man, in a brown outfit and a huge black hat that was more like a basket, scowling and gesturing and keeping up a flow of angry talk. What did I mean by lying down on the grass? Who in hell did I think I was anyway, and didn't I see the signs, "Keep off the grass"? Quickly I arose, jumped back to the cement walk and planted myself in a seat on a bench. The man did not go away. Perhaps my silence only aggravated his displeasure. He glowered with scorn and then, muttering sullenly, "Greenhorn!" he walked off. Again I asked myself, what and whom was the park for, anyway? Back in the old village not even the landlord begrudged anyone the privilege of stretching out on the grass under a birch tree in his forest. And here I could not get near a tree or grass to smell of it without inviting castigation! (That, of course, was before the days of Robert Moses and the humanization of the city parks.) Perhaps I was expecting too much of New York. But I had come from a country of grass and trees and a river abounding in water nymphs, and I yearned for an escape from the tenements, the asphalt, above all from the insufferable piles of garbage, and there was no escape.

What irked me especially was a growing sense of isolation. In spite of the crowds in the street, the ever-increasing number of boarders in our apartment to make up for the unemployment of some members of the family, in spite of the numerous friends I had made on the block, I felt cut off from the outside world, the American world, almost as completely as was our village in spring when the floods and the mud made the roads impassable. I was overcome with a boundless wish to know something of this world, touch it in person, see it, hear it, feel it, eat with it, talk with it, laugh with it, sing with it and, if it was anything like the old village emotionally, mourn and weep with it. But I did not

193

even know where to look for it. I knew it existed, a vast simmering, mysterious world, having a civilization all its own and stretching beyond New York to the Pacific Ocean, and here was I cooped up in the tenement section of the lower East Side, with not a glimmer of a chance to make its acquaintance, with hardly anyone ever speaking of it or caring for its existence.

Of course I had heard people talk of uptown. But uptown was only an extension of downtown. True, rich people lived there. The bosses, the landlords, the policemen made their homes there. No piles of garbage cluttered the streets uptown, and people there were well dressed, some of them carried canes, and everybody spoke English. Perhaps that was where real America began. I wondered and wondered. But uptown was forbidding. I might freely walk the streets there, look into windows of shops and homes, watch the endless crowds saunter up and down the avenues, and that was all. There was no way I might participate in the life there and come to know people in their intimate setting, as friends, as members of a family, as plain human beings. I could learn of them no more than what I might see with my physical eyes. Then something happened that made the very word "uptown" anathema.

I discovered the Educational Alliance, and I often went there to spend my leisure in the library reading room. I had never seen so many shelves of books in any one place, and I loved to take an armful of them, sit at the table and turn the pages. One evening a new librarian came to work there. She was a slender, gray-haired lady with tight lips and exquisitely dressed. When she saw me bring an armful of books to the table, she came over and asked why I took so many books at once. In my imperfect English I explained that I loved to look at them, turn the pages, examine illustrations and read isolated passages. After watching me in indecision for a few minutes, she went back to her desk. I didn't like her sullen look and hoped she would never again come near me. Presently she was back by my side. "Sit up straight, please," she ordered. Startled, I looked at her with protesting eyes. I had not been aware how I was sitting, and now that she had made me conscious of it, I wondered what difference it made to her. However, with no word of rejoinder I obeyed. She went away, and

194

while playing with the books I soon forgot myself and again leaned my head on my elbow. In an instant she was back at my side. "I told you to sit up straight." This time I refused to obey. I continued to turn the pages and refrained from looking at her. Again she repeated her order in a louder voice, and the boys and girls at my table looked up as if expecting trouble.

"I like it better this way," I finally growled.

"You've got to sit up straight," she ordered stiffly.

Was I tearing up the books? No. Was I breaking or scratching up the table? No. Was I calling her names? No. Why then did she demand that I sit in a position which I disliked? Incensed with her arbitrariness, I shoved the books off the table to the floor and dashed out of the room. Now I knew that the things I had heard about people uptown were true. Haughty and domineering, they didn't like the poor people downtown, and their attendant in a library reading room wouldn't even permit an immigrant boy to sit in comfort. I pronounced an ugly curse on her and hoped I should never again cross her path. To make sure of it, I never went back to that reading room, and I decided that uptown was not real America, anyway.

Soon afterwards a model came to work in the shop in which I had found a new job. Every morning when I cleaned the show-room—wiped the furniture, the racks, the mirrors—she would be there, and now and then she asked me to hang up coats which she had been exhibiting the evening before. Tall, blue-eyed, with blonde hair, she spoke in a soft voice and with an intonation that was markedly different from that which I had been hearing down-town—that is, in the section in which I lived. Whenever she asked me to do something she thanked me and smiled, not the brittle thin-lipped smile of the librarian in the Educational Alli-ance but the amiable smile of a person who liked people and wanted them to like her. Again and again I wished I had the courage to tell her that she was the most beautiful girl I had ever known. She too came from uptown, and I wondered what manner of person she was outside of the shop. Was she reading Herbert Spencer and George Eliot and going to lectures like those Ed-ward King was delivering? She was not as approachable as Lina, and I would never think of trying out my newly acquired words

195

on her as I did on Lina, but it was exhilarating to watch her move gracefully about the showroom and to hear her speak and laugh as she and a buyer bantered each other.

Now I knew that there were beautiful women uptown, and not only beautiful but gracious and kind.

I had been in the country about a year when I felt that I knew English well enough to enter high school. Some of the boys in the neighborhood counseled me to enroll in the school which they were attending, the Stuyvesant High School. A new term was about to begin, and I went to see the principal.

His name was Dr. Frank Rollins, and as I sat in the reception room waiting my turn to see him I felt anxious and agitated. To me the principal of an American high school was like the director of a Russian Gymnasium, a man of eminence and with a forbidding dignity. I therefore wondered if Dr. Rollins would grant my petition. I had not attended grammar school in this country, and technically I was not qualified for admission to high school without an examination, though the school from which I had graduated in Russia embraced a curriculum that was scholastically about the same as that of an American grammar school. The chief difference was that I had studied Russian instead of American history. I was prepared to take the examination but feared I might not pass it. In that event would "the mister director" enroll me as a trial student? In Russia he would not, but then—this was not Russia. I prayed that in the presence of the man I might not feel so agitated and confused that I would slip up in my English, which of course would at once disqualify me for admission.

I trembled all over as I went into Dr. Rollins' private office. As soon as I entered he greeted me amiably and pointed to a seat beside his own. The unexpected friendly greeting set me immediately at ease. A handsome, athletic man of about fifty, with dark hair, an expressive face and a broad smile, there was nothing in Dr. Rollins' appearance or manner that suggested the director of a Gymnasium. No ornate uniform, no social stiffness, no superimposed dignity. In no way did he make me feel that he was an official. He might have been my uncle whom I was seeing for the first time in my life, so unassuming and comradely was his

196

manner. He asked me a number of questions about myself and my life in a Russian village and about the schooling I had had in Russia. He seemed so keenly interested in my answers that he made no effort to bring the conversation to a hasty end, though I knew that many other callers were waiting in the reception room. Then, passing a sheet of paper to me and vacating his own chair so that I could sit at his desk, he asked me to write out a few of the things I had been telling him so that he could judge whether or not my written English was good enough to enable me to pursue my studies. Encouraged by his friendliness, I quickly filled the paper with writing and showed it to him. He seemed pleased and made out an admission card and told me to come the following Monday, when the new term would start. Before I left he asked if I had already decided on the profession for which I wished to prepare myself, and without an instant's hesitation I replied, "I hope to be a farmer." He laughed a little, not, I am sure, in disapproval, probably only in surprise that a student in a city high school, especially in New York, should choose farming as a career. On leaving he shook my hand and asked me to come in and see him after I had attended classes for a few weeks and tell him how I liked the American school.

My head swam with triumph. I was actually admitted to an American Gymnasium, and it was all so easy; no questions about the financial and social status of the family, no lengthy application blanks to fill out, no need to pay any tuition fees or even to buy books, and "the mister director" such an amiable and fatherly man! Here was something exciting to write about to floundering schoolmates in far-away Russia.

The students in the school came from all the boroughs of the city, and here for the first time I was beginning to rub shoulders with boys who obviously belonged to *the* America that lay culturally if not geographically somewhere beyond uptown. They wore better clothes than I did, and they were much more articulate and boisterous. They seemed completely attuned to the school and all its activities, while I with my burden of uncertainties felt out of harmony with the spirit of the place. I watched my schoolmates with curiosity and envy.

197

At first I thought that they were an extravagant horde of young barbarians. They ate a prodigious amount of sweets, cakes, pies, chocolates and other candies, and the sandwiches that they brought from home for their lunches were wrapped in spotlessly white tissue paper, each sandwich in a separate sheet. On removing the paper from the food, they rolled it together and flung it at each other or into the wastebasket. Every day the wastebaskets were stuffed with endless sheets of soft paper which would have been a luxury of luxuries to the smokers in the old village. As poor a man as Trofim the Hawk would gladly have exchanged a freshly laid egg for a bundle of the precious sheets that were to be hauled off with the garbage. Had I not been abashed, I should have gathered them in a bundle and taken them home, though what I should have done with it I knew neither then nor now. If the old village were within reaching distance I might have sent it there, and even the women who never smoked would have acclaimed it with joy.

The family finances were so low that, unless I made my contribution to the budget, I could not attend school. Luckily I found a job as errand boy and shipping clerk in a shop that needed my services only afternoons. I was glad of the job, and yet wished I could do without it so that I could participate in or at least witness some of the extracurricular activities. The whole world of athletics had been a closed book to me. From the moment I entered school I knew that basketball, baseball, football, track, were as essential and even more eloquent a part of school life than were books and classes. The lusty cheering practices were abundant testimony to the excitement of the students over athletic games. I understood neither the aims nor the intoxication of that frenzied and rhythmic yelling. Try as I might, I could not make myself a part of it. It just was not in me, and because I was occupied in the shop every afternoon, I could not burn with the fires of devotion which seemed to scorch the very benches on which the other students sat. I envied them, and yet their impassioned ra-ra-ra's gave me unending amusement. Here was something of real America of which neither beggars nor Blind Sergey had ever dreamed.

Meanwhile the work, the study, the crowded condition of our apartment, the incessant wrangles with two brothers who objected to my keeping on the gaslight in the kitchen—in which I prepared my homework and in which the three of us slept—later than their bedtime had shattered my health. I went to see Dr. Rollins, and he sent me to a clinic. Then began a series of medical examinations and pronouncements which only preyed on my mind and further devastated my health. Nerve-racked and angry at the whole world, I lost interest in school, in work, in play, and I loathed the sight of a thermometer, a stethoscope or any other medical paraphernalia.

Often I wished I were back in the old village. In spite of its mud, its miseries, its idiocies, there were trees and grass there and immense fields over which I could wander and on which I could shake off physical aches and languors and the bitterness of my soul.

Then, one day as I was on my way home from the clinic, an inner voice whispered, "Why don't you go to an American village?" Why not, indeed? The more I thought of it the more hopeful and excited I became. Eventually I was hoping to leave New York anyway. I was only waiting until I had completed my course in high school. I had set my mind and heart on an agricultural career—through college and to a farm of my own. I had two more years of high school. But then this was not Russia. I should find a high school in an American village, and I could continue my studies and go to college there, and meanwhile I should be striking roots in the American soil. More, I should be living in real America, not uptown, but 'way beyond, in the America that had intrigued and mystified and beckoned to me, but which I had neither seen nor felt nor absorbed. There would not only be trees and brooks and meadows and a real river there, but people like Blind Sergey and Amelko the Screamer—like them and yet different, of course, because after all this was America, and its monumental energy alone stirred an inner vigor and lushness which the old village with its age-old inertia and lethargy never could bring into being. I could work in this village. I was not bedridden, though I might be if I remained in New York and kept pounding my way from one clinic to another. A hoe, a

199

scythe, a plow would take the place of the tonics, the cathartics, the emetics and all the other pharmacopoeia with which I had been drenching myself, and if, because of the weakened condition of heart, lungs, nerves, I were to die, I should at least take leave of the world with my eyes not on an ugly tenement wall and a pile of garbage but on a meadow, an orchard, a stream. Back to the village, to an American village, became the slogan, the hope, the passion of my life.

CHARLES REZNIKOFF

Charles Reznikoff was born on August 31, 1894, in Brooklyn, the son of Nathan and Sarah Yetta (Wolvovsky) Reznikoff. He received his LL.B. degree from the Law School of New York University in 1915 and was admitted to the Bar of the State of New York the next year. He married Marie Syrkin in 1930 and has been managing editor of the *Jewish Frontier* since 1955.

He has written poetry, history, fiction and autobiography. He edited the public papers of Louis Marshall and translated from the German I. J. Benjamin's *My Three Years in America—1859–1862*. Among his works are *Five Groups of Verse* (1927); *Nine Plays* (verse, 1927); *By the Waters of Manhattan* (novel, 1930); *Jerusalem, the Golden* (verse, 1933); *Testimony* (prose, 1934); *The Early History of a Sewing-Machine Operator* (1936); *Separate Way* (verse, 1936); *Going To and Fro and Walking Up and Down* (verse, 1941); *The Lionhearted* (novel, 1944); *The Jews of Charlestown* (history, 1950); *Inscriptions 1944–1956* (verse); *By the Waters of Manhattan* (selected poems, 1962).

Mr. Reznikoff has never practiced law although licensed to do so. He has devoted his whole life to literature and whatever he does is characterized by meticulously fine workmanship. He is constitutionally incapable of producing hackwork. His work has never yet received its proper due in my estimation, as a number of reviews I have written in the *New Leader*, *Midstream* and *Commentary* have insisted. Over the years, his work has won some substantial admirers. Among these can be counted the imagist poet John Gould Fletcher, Lionel Trilling, Louis Untermeyer (who wrote an Introduction to the novel *By the Waters of Manhattan*), Kenneth Burke (who wrote an Introduction to the volume *Testimony*), C. P. Snow (who wrote an Introduction to his volume of selected poems, published by New Directions, for which he adopted his own earlier title *By the Waters of Manhattan*), and the poet Louis Zukofsky. His work has had some influential detractors as well, it is perhaps only fair to add. Marius Bewley, in one of his books, has a scathing notice of Reznikoff, whom he mentions in the course of a more extended attack upon Kenneth Burke. But on the principle enunciated by Oscar Wilde that the only thing worse than being talked about is not being talked about, Mr. Bewley has possibly served Reznikoff better than have all those who have failed to mention his existence at all. This includes such a vast and potent majority in the literary world of our time that Reznikoff's name is absent from virtually all the standard reference books, which should include him.

At the present time, he is launched upon the most ambitious project of his literary career. He proposes to give an impressionistic account of what it was like to live in the United States between the years 1885 and 1910 in *five* volumes of what he calls "recitative" (to distinguish it, I suppose, from verse on the one hand and prose on the other). The first of these has appeared under the title *Testimony* (a title which he also used before, in the 1930's) and has drawn some attention, both favorable and unfavorable. The poet Hayden Carruth, who had been very enthusiastic about the volume of selected poems of Reznikoff which had appeared in 1962, gave this latest book a very bad review in *Poetry* (Chicago). On the other hand, Reznikoff's work has been making friends in some of the more fashionable poets and literary people of a much younger generation than his own: Robert Creeley, May Swenson, David Ignatow, Geoffrey Woolf, Cynthia Ozick. Reznikoff has received some encouragement and signs of recognition on the West Coast of the U.S., especially in San Francisco. Perhaps this portends a new interest in his work, which it would be a misnomer to label a revival, because there has never been a sufficiently lively or widespread interest in it before. He has made his appeal to scattered individuals in the past and may continue to do so in the future as well, hopefully to more individuals rather than less as time goes by. As I think of him, I recall the consolation which Felix Adler once attempted to give to Walt Whitman, who complained not infrequently of the paucity in the number of his admirers. "Readers must not only be counted," Adler said to Whitman, "they must be weighed!" Some of Reznikoff's readers and encouragers have certainly been weighty men themselves, yet it is discouraging to note how little impression even such people have been able to make upon "the Establishment" (whatever and wherever that is), not to speak of the public at large. A standard reference book to which I have had occasion to refer, *Twentieth Century Authors*, by Kunitz and Haycroft, does not, in Reznikoff's seventy-fifth year, have any allusion to his work. It is as if he did not exist at all. Yet that book has room for a sizable article about Michael Gold and a picture of him; it describes him as "the dean of proletarian writers in the United States." It may be that Gold belongs in such a compilation, but so too, it seems to me, does Reznikoff, whose prose *By the Waters of Manhattan* appeared in the same year as Gold's *Jews Without Money* (1930) and seems to me altogether a finer, more sensitive, more interesting and durable aesthetic work. To test this, one has only to compare the texture of the passages from Reznikoff that I have included in this anthology with that of Gold's work, which has not been printed here but which is readily available since it has been reprinted in a widely circulated paperback edition.

By the Waters of Manhattan

Ezekiel reached the stoop of the tenement in which he lived and entered the dark, familiar smell. The janitor's wife—to ward off her trouble she had clothed herself in layers and balloons of fat—was floundering on the stairs like a mammal out of the deep sea. She threw an angry glance after Ezekiel as his feet left stains on the newly washed wood. "Can I help it?" he apologized.

"A nice time to come home—in the middle of the day." And she went on scrubbing, muttering curses she would not have uttered a syllable of, if there were any likelihood of their coming true.

Ezekiel was glad to find that his mother was not at home. His two brothers, too young to go to school, were playing on the floor with pots and pans dragged out of the kitchen closet. The younger, just then, was sitting disconsolately in a pool. Ezekiel searched for the scrubbing brush and wrapped it in a newspaper together with a box of scouring powder and a bar of yellow soap (that had been washed from its pristine square into a smooth, matronly waistline). With these under his arm he passed the janitor's wife, who had now reached the tiles of the two-by-four vestibule.

Then he saw that he had forgotten rags to use as a mop—and a pail would be handy. He went back, put everything in the pail and wrapped that in the newspaper, a bundle no longer as genteel as at first.

He hurried towards the store. Now and then he felt for the key in his pocket. Why hadn't he eaten when he was at home? He was

Selections from Charles Reznikoff's *By the Waters of Manhattan*, published by Charles Boni, New York, 1930.

weak and shaky. Well, he wouldn't go back. He walked another block and a half. It was no use. He must eat, otherwise he wouldn't have strength to do the cleaning. And he had forgotten the broom. Couldn't he have sat down calmly and thought out all that he needed instead of snatching up a few things, and then hurrying back and snatching up a few things more?

His mother would be home by this time. She would come in and see the mess on the floor, put down her bags and bundles, catch up the youngsters and give them a few slaps. Then she would look for a rag to wipe the floor, and find the rags gone and the pail gone—he smiled at her bewilderment.

But when he got home, his mother had not yet come. He lit the gas and put the kettle on, and cut himself a thick slice of black bread. His brothers at once set up a yell for bread and he cut them each a slice. He began eating his slowly, waiting for the kettle to boil.

How good the bread tasted. He studied the smooth, brown upper crust and the thick under crust, white with flour. How good it was. He ate thankfully and understood how men have come to say grace.

The door opened. His mother came in, a bulging market bag hanging from her hand. "Oh, Zecky, I'm so glad you're home. I forgot potatoes—and to climb the stairs again. Hurry up, Zecky. It's late already. And look what they did here!" She raised her voice at the sight of the pots and pans and the trail of the young-ster with soaking rompers.

Ezekiel was about to protest. He had his own work to do. But at the sight and sound of her anger at the children, he held out his hand for the nickel and pennies.

On his way back he thought, Now I'll have to tell Ma what I want the things for. There's so much to explain and nothing may come of it. Ezekiel was afraid that if he told, somehow his strength would ooze away. And he liked to think that in these apparently aimless wanderings, he was working out an intricate and beautiful design. He would simply tell his mother that he needed the soap and things, that he would bring them right back, and would explain afterwards.

He put the bag of potatoes on the washtub. His brothers, tears still in their eyes from the spanking, jumped about, shouting, "I wanna napple, I wanna napple." The bag fell to one side and out of its curves rolled two or three potatoes. At their dismal brown, the noise stopped. "Zecky, I haven't a match in the house," his mother began plaintively.

It would have been easy enough to borrow some next door, if the people had not moved out. The walk to his store would take him forty minutes. It would soon be dark, and what could he do there then? "What is the matter with you?" he shouted. "My whole day is taken up running around for you. Can't you tell me everything at one time?"

"Well, I forgot. Believe me, I have enough on my head. Am I playing? Don't you see I haven't got a minute's rest? And I have lived to have a son like you—a help! Not a penny does he bring in the house, but give him eat, give him clothes, and he bosses yet. A blessing on our heads! And when I ask him to run down for me a minute, when I am so tired I can't stand on my feet, look at the mouth he opens. Have you heard it?"

"All right, all right, I'll go, I'll go, only keep still."

"Go in the hell! Here." She counted three pennies out of her pocketbook and slapped them on the table. He picked them up and ran downstairs.

His mother thought, as she peeled the potatoes and they fell white and plump into the clear water, What is the matter with my head that I forget like that? He is right. Is it right to send a man to the grocery like a little boy? I must make him think himself a man with a man's work to do, and I keep treating him like a boy. Is it any wonder that he acts like he does?

It was too late to go to his store. In a little while it began to grow dark. From the window, Ezekiel saw the peddlers taking their places along the curb. Soon the sidewalks, and the gutters, too, were crowded with working men and girls going home. The peddlers shouted. Three or four pushcarts had gas-jets, now flaring the twilight. The shop windows and electric signs lit up. Ezekiel heard the purring of the sign below. It was night at last. In the street the peddlers shouted. Ezekiel heard the elevated trains, the clanging streetcars, the impatient horns of the motor trucks, the thousand feet and voices of the crowd at high tide.

The gas was lit in the kitchen. He saw his sisters moving about. As Ezekiel went in, the light hurt his eyes.

His father was seated at the table and on a plate before him were two potatoes, smoking hot. As he broke them up and swallowed piece after piece, Saul kept opening his thick lips and drawing in his breath to cool the lump of potato, his mouth and throat. Like a fish, Ezekiel thought.

Ezekiel's sisters were bringing plates to the table and talking to each other. "Cut bread," their mother shouted, bending over the pot.

"You do it," Esther shouted at her sister, "don't you see I'm setting the table?"

"And what am I doing, you dope?"

Their father banged the table with his fist so that the plates and cutlery jumped. "Let it be still," he shouted in Yiddish. "Enough noise all day in the shop. When I come home, I want quiet."

They were silent. He fell to on the meat and potatoes heaped upon his plate. The sisters made faces at each other. Sarah Yetta served her daughters and son, darting angry glances at each.

When he had finished, Saul slouched back, his head sunk forward, his eyes fixed in a stare. Ezekiel studied their yellowish whites with specks of red and blue and the faded brown of the pupils. The bald forehead, breaking out in a fine sweat, glistened under the gaslight. His cheeks and chin were covered with a brown and grey bristle.

A belch shook him. He got up slowly and walked to the sink, spat into it and poured himself a glass of water. "Why don't we have water on the table?" he said crossly, and went into the bedroom.

They could hear the bed creak as he sat on it. And then the shoes hit the floor, one, two. The bed creaked again, and all was still.

Esther had put on her hat and with her little finger was smearing the red of the lipstick over her lips. "Where are you going?" Rebecca whispered in agony. "It's your turn to wash the dishes. It ain't fair, Ma, it ain't fair."

"I don't feel well tonight," Esther said, and turned on Ezekiel. "Why don't you do it? We work hard all day. You don't do nothing, why don't you do it? I'm not going to do it, let him do it." And she hurried out, closing the door behind her against argument and threat.

"Yes," Rebecca took up the attack, "we work hard all day. We got enough to do."

"Keep still, you'll wake up the children, you'll wake Papa up. I don't want him to do it. It isn't a man's work. I'll do it myself." And Sarah Yetta rose and began piling up the dishes.

"I don't want you to, Mamma," Rebecca said, "go away." And she began to carry the dishes to the sink. Her eyes overflowed. "But it ain't fair, Mamma, it ain't fair. It's Esther's turn tonight. And, anyway, Zecky ought to do it. He don't do nothing all day now. Why can't he do it, the big bum?" Ezekiel took his cap and went out.

The stoop was empty. If it were summer it would be crowded and he thought of himself picking his way among those seated along the steps. Excuse me. There! He had stepped on someone's hand. He could feel the fingers numb between his shoe and the stone.

He crossed the Bowery and walked up Prince Street, through the Italian quarter. The street was quiet. A wall of red brick shut in the garden of a nunnery, all but an elm that managed to look over. Broadway, too, was quiet: just a man or a motor car, now and then, and a streetcar, almost empty. The side streets were black, except where the lamps lit up the shop signs and the silence.

At last he came to his store. The shine of the street lamps along the plate glass—the window seemed to him a pool in the desert of brick houses. He tried to look inside, but all was pitch dark.

Should he open the door and go in? To do what in the darkness? He took out the key. He would just try the lock.

He slipped the key into the keyhole and imagined himself a thief. He tried to turn the key gently. It would not budge. For a panic-stricken minute he pressed hard upon it, the bolt slid back with a loud noise, and the door was open. Then he turned the key back and tried the handle three or four times to make sure the door was locked.

His mother and sisters would still be up. The kitchen, in which he slept, would be crowded with their talk—to fall on his mind like handfuls of gravel on a pane of glass. He walked along the streets, imagining them canals and bathing in their silence.

He became impatient, wanted the night done with as soon as possible, thought of all the days he had wasted, and stretched out for the morrow. It was early and the street in which he lived was still noisy.

He opened the door. Yes, his mother and Rebecca were seated in the glare of the gaslight, talking away. "Listen, I've got to go to bed early," he said, "so please go out."

"What's the matter, you've got a job?" Rebecca sneered. They had long given up hope of any job for Ezekiel. What to do with him was a mountain in their midst, at which they each shied an angry or malicious or calmly earnest word, but the mountain stayed.

"Go on out now. Mamma, I've got to get up early. Go down to the stoop if you want to talk. Anyway, what are you staying cooped up here for?"

His mother went into the bedroom. "It's too early to go to bed," Rebecca said. "Only people who don't have to work go to bed now," and she slammed the door behind her.

Ezekiel ran after her into the hall to punch her. "Do you want to wake up Papa and the kids?" She screamed, and catching hold of the banisters, clattered downstairs.

His mother had brought out his quilts, sheet, and pillow. "Don't bother, Ma." He pushed the chairs together to make his bed on them.

She stood in the doorway. "What's a matter, Zecky? Don't you feel good? Does your head hurt?"

"I've got a lot of work tomorrow and I want to go to bed early. I feel fine, Ma. Good-night."

The light of the window across the airshaft covered him with a golden cloth. The distant noises of the street and the dim voices of the neighbors, his father's snoring, the faint noises that his mother made beyond the closed door as she undressed, fell silently into his calm spirit.

His steps became slow. In the daylight how drab his plans were.

He saw the sun large as it is, not small as it seems, and the earth, small as it is, not large as it seems. What men have done and what a man, if he were to meet a being of another planet, might boast of, seemed to him at that moment unimportant, as the earth itself in the heavens.

He was tired, as if his muscles were tired. If the grave were open, he would step in, to be out of the noise of the world and its lights, the great light and the lesser lights and the many tiny lights that man has made, to rest in the darkness, in the black of nothingness forever.

The wind blew the dust of the street into his face, blackening his nostrils, blew dust upon his lips. How should he escape? From how many windows and roofs to fall, before how many trains, cars, and motor cars to jump, how easy to walk into the Harlem River, the East River, the Hudson River, the Bay, the Sound, the sea at a hundred beaches.

Why should he? Surely he who cared so little for life could dare heights and distances—there to find, perhaps, nectar and ambrosia? So after all I am a romanticist, Ezekiel thought.

Now his wish to live ordered him into action. And like a good private, without further question, sure of no other value in the command but to make him forget himself, he came home quickly to do what he had planned.

Why should I keep it a secret, he thought, if it would give Ma a little courage about me? So he told her what he had done and wanted to do.

She looked at him doubtfully. She had heard too many of his plans and had seen them come to nothing. But she gave him what he asked for. "Bring them right back, soon as you are through." When the door closed behind him, she went to the window and said a little prayer.

Ezekiel turned the faucet of the sink in the back of the store. For a moment he was afraid that the water was shut off, but it splashed down with a cheerful noise. He took its presence as a good omen and imagined himself one of his ancestors who had just dug a well in the desert.

He filled the pail and set to work scrubbing the floor. This was only covered with dust; it was no hard job to make the floor fairly clean again. As he was kneeling over the scrubbing brush and the bubbling wash it left, he heard the door opened. The grocer looked on, smiling. "Hard at it, eh?"

It was a long time since he had seen approval in anybody's eyes and a stranger's at that. Ezekiel worked with a will. It was pleasant to have a job after his long idleness, pleasant to move his muscles, pleasant to make the dirty floor clean, the dirty window shine, to rub the woodwork clean of dust, and to know, when all was done, he would be the master.

At last he was through. An empty box had been left in the store and he stood this up for a seat. He washed his hands and waved them in the air until they were dry. Then he took out of his pocket the piece of rye bread he had brought with him, and seated on the box ate slowly, gazing with satisfaction at the wet floor and bright window.

He was tired; his knees ached and his arms ached. Though he had started briskly enough, when he had gone a little way, he slowed up and the walk home never seemed as long and tedious and the stairs as troublesome. He placed his bundle on the wash-tub and felt that he could do no more that day.

He walked to the front room and sat in the armchair. He thought of his shop, the clean floor on which the water was drying and the bright window. He remembered how, too young to walk, he was crawling up a dark flight of stairs. Upon the upper landing the sunlight shone through a window.

His mother came gently into the room. She smiled and said, "You are not used to that work. Lie down a little." She wiped an apple in her apron until the red skin shone, and left it on the arm of the chair.

He held the apple to his nose. He had read of a dying rabbi who kept smelling at an apple for the strength to speak his last words. Bright and red, it was the earth upon which the sun shone. It seemed to Ezekiel that the world was good and every breath he drew precious. His body was tired, but his heart fresh and joyful.

To pass the time he wondered what he would do if he had a nickel. He might buy a cup of coffee or a bar of chocolate or a box of crackers or a roll and two penny packages of chocolate or

211

an apple and a roll or a loaf of bread. It was ridiculous to be in want of just a nickel in the streets of New York.

When he was a boy, he sometimes found a penny—once a dime—in the streets. Surely there were hundreds and hundreds of dollars in change lying that moment along the miles of sidewalks and in the gutters. If he were to devote himself to looking for it, he might make a good living and, certainly, it was not as unpleasant as some work. He would be in the open air, at least.

If a coin should drop on the sidewalk, it would be quickly picked up. But if money fell out of men's pockets as they hurried across the street, Ezekiel reasoned, it would roll into the gutters. The street-cleaners, most likely, picked up everything there: between their rounds was his chance. He saw himself a savage hunting for a root he knew of to stop his hunger. If there was woodcraft, Ezekiel thought, he was master of a new science, citycraft.

He began to search at once, walking along the curb, his eyes in the gutter. Now and then he could not help stepping off and so often an automobile or truck rushed close by, he realized the business was not without its dangers. After only a block and a half he found a quarter. There it was, shiny in the newly swept gutter, the marks of the street-cleaner's broom across it. He picked it up and looked about.

The quarter was worn smooth and he let it clink on the sidewalk to make sure it was not counterfeit. He was too impatient now for anything but a restaurant. At an Automat, five or six blocks down, he changed it into real nickels, and smiled at the thought that the cashier might say, "This quarter is no good: ' 'tis of the unsubstantial fabric of a dream.' "

This was going to be a feast and for that he would wash his hands carefully. Though he was so hungry, now that he would be fed, he took his time. He delighted in the cool water and the rough clean paper towels. Then he made the round of the little compartments and studied through the thick glass the little pots of dark brown beans, the meat pies—the brown crust curling away from the thick dishes—the dishes of macaroni with yellow nuggets of melted cheese, the pompous apple dumplings in ermine of vanilla sauce, then the sandwiches: rows bright with

212

sliced tomatoes and green lettuce, with the red of smoked meats, or the pastel tints of cheese.

Why spend anything? He was going home. He would weaken himself not only by having less, but in that he yielded. Still, to spend one nickel would not be extravagant, and he ought to celebrate.

Coffee streamed into his cup. He lowered his head to breathe its fragrance. It seemed to him that he was carrying a small pot of earth from which the steam, a fragrant bush, grew. The grains of sugar in the heaping teaspoonful glittered. They sank into the coffee and their light became sweetness. He drank slowly.

It warmed and cheered him. The lights of the ceiling shone into the core of his being. He thought of himself as a soldier, resting from battle, or a sailor, during a lull in the storm, drinking hot coffee.

He walked for a block or two before he remembered to look along the gutter. For a mile he found nothing. A policeman eyed him. At last he picked up a dime. It was no longer precious and he looked no more.

In the Italian quarter he joined a crowd before a florist's shop. Out came the picture of a saint on the shoulders of bare-headed men, the frame stuck over with pink paper roses and green dollar bills. The brass band in the middle of the street struck up a lively air, most of the men in the crowd took off their hats, the open windows of the tenements were jammed with women and children. First went the band, then the sacred picture with a guard of children in Sunday clothes, their tall yellow candles burning strangely in the sunlight, then a red banner and the men of its society.

The procession turned into a street hung with arches of colored electric bulbs and made its way between the pushcarts and crowd until it reached a little red church. There the band played louder than ever, a priest came to the porch to welcome the picture and it was brought inside; the worshippers and their lighted candles followed. Women from neighboring houses, covering their heads with black shawls, hurried to join them.

Ezekiel waited in the street. As they came down the steps, the men who carried the picture were sweating under the heavy frame. He studied their stolid faces. The priest was left on the steps. Still a young man, his fat belly showed under the cassock; his ruddy face with its high broad forehead was proud and intelligent.

The procession was on its way back. As he kept his hands raised blessing it, the priest lifted his eyes to a window across the street. Ezekiel followed his glance and saw over a flowerbox a face as intelligent as the priest's, but it was thin; the man had long black hair, and his lips were curled in a broad smile. Beside him stood a woman and her ruddy, pretty face was also wreathed in smiles. The priest turned to the procession and its crowd, now half way up the block, and flung his hands down as if in disgust. He smiled up to the smiling man and woman.

The comedy over, Ezekiel walked the gallery of the pushcarts, examining the exhibits: the peaceful colors of vegetables or a cart bright with oranges. When he came to a Carnegie library, he went in out of habit. It seemed to him a long time since he had been in such a room. He took an anthology from the shelf and read a page here and there. The lights were lit and still he read on.

When he was back in the street it was night. He was cold and faint with hunger. He opened the door and found them all about the table. As he ate his eyes closed for weariness. He would have gone to sleep as soon as dinner was over, but the dishes had to be washed and wiped and put away and the room would be noisy and lighted for a long time.

It was too cold to sleep on the roof. He spread his blanket at the end of the hall: they lived on the top floor and no one would be going to the roof now. He took off his shoes and put them alongside; untied his necktie and stuffed it into his pocket, and unbuttoned the collar of his shirt. Surely a necktie, he thought, is Jeremiah's halter that a man ties about his neck each day as a symbol of his life.

How good to rest. The gas-jet in the hall on the floor below was lit: how pleasant to lie in the darkness and see the light streaming up between the banisters. He heard a squabble in his home. It did not matter: he was outside. Soon the oil of sleep pouring over him drowned his mind.

Something had touched his face. It was pitch dark: after ten o'clock the light downstairs was out. He caught up the blanket to go into the house. Something soft fell on the floor and scampered away, its nails faintly clicking. Too light for a dog or cat and too heavy for a mouse. A rat! He shivered and felt his upper lip curl in disgust.

It was cold in the kitchen, too. It was too early in the season to make the stove; for it was only cold late at night when everyone was or ought to be asleep and covered. He was stiff and knocked into a chair. He felt about in the dark, put the chairs together, undressed, then spread the blanket on the seats and wrapping himself in it, with his arm for a pillow, fell asleep.

He was walking in a narrow street and after a while knew it as the stable street through which he went to kindergarten. The large doors of the stables were open, for it was May. In the dark interiors he could sometimes see a man polishing a carriage or leading a horse with noisy hoofs up an incline. The stench of the stables burned his nostrils, but in his hand was a spray of lilacs. This was for his teacher. He bent over to smell the lilacs only. A cluster touched his face. It was like the muzzle of the rat and he woke with a start.

The sky was grey. The dawn lit up the kitchen and he was wide awake (because he had gone to sleep so early the night before). He hurried to dress and wash and be out under that strange sky before it was day.

No one was in the street but the milkman. Lights were shining in the groceries: he could see the grocers and their sleepy boys filling paper bags with rolls, the warm smell of which filtered through the open doors.

Ezekiel took deep breaths of the cold air. Even these streets were quiet now. His sleep had become a long pleasant dream. In the bright morning he looked eagerly at the houses, at each horse and milkwagon—some had the lantern hung from the axle still burning—and at each vivid laborer that passed.

More and more people were in the streets, until Ezekiel, thinking of Wordsworth, found himself in the light of common day.

He felt for the four nickels in his pocket. The silver of the thin dime was an unexpected pleasure: he had not thought of it and it was as if he had just found it. He would not have to go home for breakfast; and this taste of freedom was so dear to him, he made up his mind to husband every cent he could to be free.

He reached the Automat where he had had coffee the afternoon before. Now a row of compartments showed halves of melons, gaudy reddish yellows, and at the steam table were strips of bacon, dark against a huge dish of scrambled eggs. He had coffee and the modest yellow of three corn muffins, and was satisfied.

He had planned to ask the grocer for empty boxes and set them together as a table. This would have to do for fixtures, except two boxes he would use to sit on, until he had money to spend on shelving and a real table and chairs. He had better wait, though, until the shipment of books came before asking for the boxes.

There were other publishers he was now eager to see, but the delivery man from Diamond's must not find the door closed. Ezekiel took two of his own books and placed them as a seat on the cold stone of the step.

He turned to the poem James of Scotland wrote when a prisoner in the Tower of London. The *King's Quair* was fresh and pleasant in the early morning: the garden, trees and flowers, and birds singing, and the three ladies with their fresh fair faces walking along the path beside the hedge. He read on along the even rise and fall of the rich rhyme, until a shadow covered the page.

He looked up at a girl, a twinkle in her blue eyes the brighter for her dark skin.

"Are you the owner?"

"Yes," he said.

"Well, what have you for sale?" And she looked into the empty store with a mischievous smile.

"Won't you come in and see?" he said gravely, picking up the two books in the way. The King sang on and Ezekiel felt as merry, though he kept his face as grave, as the Barmecide in the *Arabian Nights*. She hesitated and then crossed the threshold.

"Here," he said, pointing to the blank wall, "are paintings from Japan. If I were an artist, I would go to Tokio, not to Paris.

216

Look," and remembering an exhibit he had seen several times, "here is a catfish turning in the water. The motion of all the waters of earth is here; here are all the ripples, currents, waves and tides; here is the horror of muddy depths of ponds, lakes, and rivers, and of the green depths of the sea, the horror of cold-blooded fish and crawling things.

"Here is a white cat under a spray of white flowers. The cat looks up at us: its body bulges, the green eyes burn among the dull whites of fur and flowers. Here are cranes on a frosty morning. The two birds, hunched up, shiver. See, about the soft, blurred white of their bodies the reeds in broad curves—grey reeds, dull green reeds, dull brown and red," and Ezekiel pointed to some cracks in the wall. "And here is a sparrow flattened against a branch for warmth. From the brown twigs hang a few brown leaves, swayed to one side by the wind. See, the polished blue-white sky of winter."

Ezekiel turned from the wall. They had reached the back of the store. "As you see, there are more, better ones, but you are tired. I'll show you the rest another time."

"I'm not tired at all. Please go on."

"I've lots besides Japanese paintings. Here is something from the Chinese. Hold one end of the scroll, please. Now," and Ezekiel made believe he was unrolling it, "look at this prairie fire. What a sweep of flames! See the little blackened skeletons of trees left behind. The flames are coming down on this field of large feathery stalks of grass. Here is a gazelle in front of the flames, its head lifted in agony. Here is the white tail of another, diving into the grass. The sky in back is golden with fire, in front black with smoke." He waved the scroll aside without troubling to roll it up.

She stood quite close to him. It seemed easy enough to put his arm about her and say, "Here's a kiss for breakfast," and he was sure she would not mind. But he had never kissed a woman and was timid. Besides, that Chinese scroll with its flames—the only one he could think of at the moment—might have put her out of the mood for kisses.

"I am going to open a bookshop," he said simply, "and I hope when the books come, you'll visit us."

217

"I'd be glad to," she said. "I see you have a few books."

"These are not for sale: they are mine." As he bent to show them, he uncovered the signs he meant to place on the window. "What do you think of these? I can't afford to have the window lettered just now. I mean to paste these up instead."

She took them from his hand. "Who is J. P. Irvine?"

"I don't think many know of him. I have never read of him anywhere, nor anything of his except in John Burroughs' anthology. What do you think of this at the end of his poem *Indian Summer?*

> The sharp staccato barking of a squirrel,
> A dropping nut, and all again is still.

Or this from *An August Afternoon on the Farm?*

> So dragged the day, but when the dusk grew deep
> The stagnant heat increased; we lit no light,
> But sat out-doors, too faint and sick for sleep."

After a minute she said, "Very good." But Ezekiel could see that her eyes were far away and the words mechanical. She shook her head slightly as if to rouse herself. "Thank you so much. I write verse myself and some day I'll come in and let you read mine." As if this could only be followed by a retreat, she added hurriedly, "I'll be late uptown," and gave him her hand.

He sat down on the steps. At noon he thought of buying a box of crackers at the landlord's but was afraid of questions, for he could still show nothing but the cleaning he himself had given the place. He scrawled a sign, "Back in two minutes," stuck it on the door, and left in a fever for fear the delivery man should come while he was out. It seemed to him many blocks before he found a grocery and he ran all the way back, half expecting to see someone waiting in front of the store.

The crackers filled his mouth with dust, but he chewed away resolutely until he had eaten all. He made a cup of his hands: the water from the faucet, even though he let it run a long time, had tiny flakes of black in it. He decided not to drink. After a while his thirst would pass, as it often did, just like hunger and cold. The body, he had found, makes its need known and after a while, unanswered, concludes its master cannot satisfy it, though he would, or is busy, and courteously becomes silent.

He wondered at the body's wisdom that is not of the mind and how each of the body's parts lives its own life. He saw himself a composite, his life a number of particles, like the mist—returning to air and water as the weather changes. Images, like frost on a window-pane, grew out of each other in his mind—to melt away.

The afternoon passed slowly. No one came in, and of those who passed, none gave the shop more than a glance. The books did not come.

How pleasantly the day had begun and how it was ending, quietly and sad, as the end of most men and women, he thought: not the "misery and madness" Wordsworth tells of as the end of poets—"we poets whose lives begin in gladness"—but such an end as Wordsworth's, plenty of money, enough milk for tea, parted from the friends of his youth, writing on and on—everything said long before, his sister's mind gone and only her smile still the same, and the sunlight, yes, even "the light of common day" fading out of the sky, little done and neither strength nor light nor time in which to do more.

Ezekiel felt his own disappointment lost in the ocean of human sorrow surging over the tallest buildings. He wondered if men, like coral, would be able to build on their own skeletons dry land at last.

He waited on until it was black night. He locked the door and was walking away, when it struck him, since bookshops were often open at night, a delivery might be made later. He turned back and waited in the darkness. He wondered, should Diamond's man come, if it were not better to have the store closed and dark than open and dark; if it would have betrayed an impatience disquieting to Mr. Diamond to have telephoned that the books had not come, or whether it showed a disquieting indifference not to have telephoned.

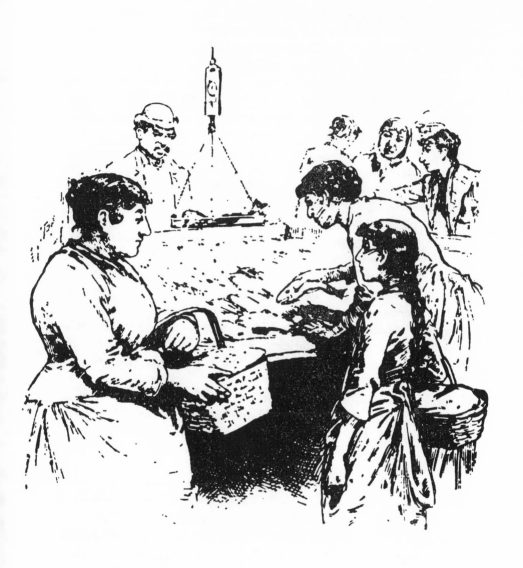

HENRY ROTH

Henry Roth is the author of one book, *Call It Sleep,* which was published in December 1934, received a number of very good notices from responsible readers and was promptly lost in the shuffle of new books. According to the author himself, its first edition numbered only 1,500 copies, its second 2,500 copies. There were no other editions until 1960, when a new, well-printed and well-bound edition in cloth came out "graced" by three separate introductions, by Harold Ribalow, Maxwell Geismar and Meyer Levin. It was greeted politely in some quarters, received scant attention in most others, was reviewed favorably by some of the same people, like Marie Syrkin, who had spoken of it glowingly before, and was certainly far from a smashing success. It was not until the paperback edition came out some years later that it appeared on the map of general public literary consciousness, became a best-seller for a time and has continued to be a very good seller ever since.

Now this is a strange literary history indeed, and the book which made this history (or helped to make it) is, as one might expect, equally strange. I feel that the last word about it is very far from having been said even yet, more than thirty years after it first appeared in the world. Is it a case of delayed recognition of indisputable artistic worth that explains its varying fortunes, like that of Melville and *Moby-Dick* (a remainder of the first edition of which could still be purchased seventy years after it was published for fifty cents!) or is it a phenomenon of a different kind with which we have to do here? To put a still more blunt question, does the book really deserve the acclaim it has received and its success in the marketplace, or are these due to high-powered public relations and advertising with which journalistic criticism and bookstore sales sometimes cross tracks? Even the putting of such questions and the call for a suspension of judgment at least until their meaning can be considered may be regarded by some persons as a very unkindly act, but that cannot be helped.

In any case, we owe a debt of gratitude to Harold Ribalow, who appears to have been primarily responsible for the 1960 edition, for the energy which he put into his research into the background of the author and the factual outline of the latter's career which he has communicated to us in his Introduction to that edition. Henry Roth was born on February 8, 1906, attended De Witt Clinton High School in New York and was graduated from the College of the City of New York in 1928. The unsettlingly contradictory reception of his work plagued him while he was an undergraduate as well as later on. He said to Ribalow: "I began to write at City College where my theme in an English course made the Year Book but I received a D in the course."

While he was at the City College, he met Eda Lou Walton, a poet and reviewer of some repute at the time who was also teaching at New York University. It was she who encouraged him to start writing *Call It Sleep*, which is dedicated to her. When the book was finished it was turned down by the first publisher to whom it was submitted, but accepted by a second. Though its sales were disappointing, the quality of the reviews and the promise displayed in a hundred-page section of a new novel by Roth "about a Communist living in the Midwest" induced Maxwell Perkins of *Scribner's* to sign the author to a new contract and to give him an advance. He never completed it.

In 1938, he went to Yaddo, where he met his wife; they lived for a while in New York. Then he spent some time on the West Coast. He returned to teach at a high school in the Bronx but soon gave this up and was able, in 1940, through a knowledge of mathematics to get a job as a machine-shop precision metal grinder—a trade with which he stayed until after the war. In 1945, he quit New York and got a job as a grinder in Cambridge, Massachusetts, where he stayed for about a year. But soon he was on the move again. He told Ribalow: "I saw by the Boston

222

newspapers that Maine real estate was very cheap. I sent my family to Montville for the summer and they liked it well enough for me to think seriously of moving to Maine and finally I did. For a year I taught school in a one-room schoolhouse and nearly went mad before the term was over. The effort was too much for me and I looked for other work because there was no need for a precision metal grinder in the state of Maine. I got a job at the Augusta State Hospital as an orderly at $26.70 a week, with room and board. I was there four years, from 1949 to 1953, and at the end of that time was a supervisor."

He bought the house he now lives in, in 1949, and his wife, as soon as the children were old enough for school, began to teach. In 1953, when he left the hospital, Roth decided to raise water-fowl, and that is his occupation now. He explained: "There's a brook behind my house which makes it rather practical. Other-wise I would never have thought of it." His conversations with Ribalow indicate his self-consciousness of the incongruity of his present mode of life and work with his whole long background: "It is odd that here I am, an East Sider, who hates to kill, in the position of slaughtering all these geese and ducks for farmers who have no compunction about killing fowl. But they haven't the time. And, after I kill the first duck of the day, I get by. But that first one is always difficult." He confessed to a period of depression in 1956 when he entered his fiftieth year, but said that the next year his interest in mathematics had revived, he began to tutor boys in the neighborhood in the subject and regained his health. Ribalow comments: "The man appeared to be at peace with himself and who was to say that obscurity on a byroad in Maine cannot lead to happiness?"

But all of these facts are more or less irrelevant to the value of that singular literary work, which is the only reason that the larger world outside has taken any interest in him at all. *Call It Sleep* is the work of a skilled verbal artificer, who shows some-thing of the same turn of mind in this field that made him a precision craftsman in another. His transposition of Yiddish speech into witty English equivalents must have required im-mense patience. At his best, he has achieved some delightful and amusing effects. The architecture of the book's overall construction seems to me less satisfactorily handled, and the ending of the book, which has been praised by some readers, is to me its weakest and most imitative section. The imitation is of James Joyce's manner of handling a stream of consciousness. Professor Rideout in his *Radical Novel in America* may be correct in calling this the best example of the "proletarian" genre, but that is only to damn with faint praise; it is to say no more than that it is the best of a bad lot.

An ecstatic review on the front page of the *New York Times Book Review* which may have launched the recent paperback reprint into popularity described *Call It Sleep* as one of the great books of the twentieth century. Such inflation seems to me to debase the critical coinage. A jaundiced eye might well conclude that Scott Fitzgerald's prejudiced prediction (in an article hailing the advent of Hemingway in the *Bookman* in 1926) of a novel that was bound to come of "the Jewish tenement block, festooned with wreaths out of *Ulysses* and the later Gertrude Stein" comes closer to the truth as an evaluation of Roth's work.

But there is no need for us to accept either of these extreme positions. The book is certainly better than the public was led to realize in the 1930's when it appeared; it is not nearly so good absolutely as some literary journalists have attempted to persuade us it is in the 1960's. It has had an impressive literary longevity, and it deserves to go on living, if only because it has undertaken to represent, both passionately and cleverly, a form of life, a kind of people, a section of America, which has had too few representations as adequate or sensitive.

Call It Sleep

One edge shining in the vanishing sunlight, the little white-washed house of the cheder lay before them. It was only one story high, the windows quite close to the ground. Its bulkier neighbors, the tall tenements that surrounded it, seemed to puff out their littered fire-escapes in scorn. Smoke curled from a little, black chimney in the middle of its roof, and overhead myriads of wash-lines criss-crossed intricately, snaring the sky in a dark net. Most of the lines were bare, but here and there was one sagging with white and colored wash, from which now and again a flurry of rinsings splashed into the yard or drummed on the cheder roof.

"I hope," said his mother, as they went down the wooden stairs that led into the yard, "that you'll prove more gifted in the ancient tongue than I was. When I went to cheder, my rabbi was always wagging his head at me and swearing I had a calf's brain." And she laughed. "But I think the reason I was such a dunce was that I could never wrench my nose far enough away to escape his breath. Pray this one is not so fond of onions!"

They crossed the short space of the yard and his mother opened the cheder door. A billow of drowsy air rolled out at them. It seemed dark inside. On their entrance, the hum of voices ceased.

The rabbi, a man in a skullcap, who had been sitting near the window beside one of his pupils, looked up when he saw them and rose. Against the window, he looked short and bulbous, oddly round beneath the square outline of the skullcap.

Selections from Henry Roth's *Call It Sleep*, first published in New York in 1934; republished by Pageant Press, Paterson, New Jersey, 1960.

"Good day," he ambled toward them. "I'm Reb Yidel Pan-
kower. You wish—?" He ran large, hairy fingers through a
glossy, crinkled beard.

David's mother introduced herself and then went on to explain
her mission.

"And this is he?"

"Yes. The only one I have."

"Only one such pretty star?" He chuckled and reaching out,
caught David's cheek in a tobacco-reeking pinch. David shied
slightly.

While his mother and the rabbi were discussing the hours and
the price and the manner of David's tuition, David scanned his
future teacher more closely. He was not at all like the teachers at
school, but David had seen rabbis before and knew he wouldn't
be. He appeared old and was certainly untidy. He wore soft
leather shoes like house-slippers, that had no place for either
laces or buttons. His trousers were baggy and stained, a great
area of striped and crumpled shirt intervened between his belt
and his bulging vest. The knot of his tie, which was nearer one
ear than the other, hung away from his soiled collar. What features were visible were large and had an oily gleam. Beneath his
skullcap, his black hair was closely cropped. Though full of misgivings about his future relations with the rabbi, David felt that
he must accept his fate. Was it not his father's decree that he
attend a cheder?

From the rabbi his eyes wandered about the room. Bare walls,
the brown paint on it full of long wavering cracks. Against one
wall, stood a round-bellied stove whose shape reminded him of
his rabbi, except that it was heated a dull red and his rabbi's
apparel was black. Against the other wall a long line of benches
ran to the rabbi's table. Boys of varying ages were seated upon
them, jabbering, disputing, gambling for various things, scuffling
over what looked to David like a few sticks. Seated upon the
bench before the rabbi's table were several others obviously waiting their turn at the book lying open in front of the rabbi's
cushioned chair.

What had been, when he and his mother had entered, a low
hum of voices, had now swollen to a roar. It looked as though

half of the boys in the room had engaged the other half in some verbal or physical conflict. The rabbi, excusing himself to David's mother, turned toward them, and with a thunderous rap of his fist against the door, uttered a ferocious, "Shah!" The noise subsided somewhat. He swept the room with angry, glittering eyes, then softening into a smile again returned to David's mother.

At last it was arranged and the rabbi wrote down his new pupil's name and address. David gathered that he was to receive his instruction somewhere between the hours of three and six, that he was to come to the cheder shortly after three, and that the fee for his education would be twenty-five cents a week. Moreover he was to begin that afternoon. This was something of an unpleasant surprise and at first he protested, but when his mother urged him and the rabbi assured him that his first lesson would not take long, he consented, and mournfully received his mother's parting kiss.

"Sit down over there," said the rabbi curtly as soon as his mother had left. "And don't forget," he brought a crooked knuckle to his lips. "In a cheder one must be quiet."

David sat down, and the rabbi walked back to his seat beside the window. Instead of sitting down, however, he reached under his chair, and bringing out a short-thonged cat-o'-nine-tails, struck the table loudly with the butt-end and pronounced in a menacing voice: "Let there be a hush among you!" And a scared silence instantly locking all mouths, he seated himself. He then picked up a little stick lying on the table and pointed to the book, whereupon a boy sitting next to him began droning out sounds in a strange and secret tongue.

For awhile, David listened intently to the sound of the words. It was Hebrew, he knew, the same mysterious language his mother used before the candles, the same his father used when he read from a book during the holidays—and that time before drinking wine. Not Yiddish, Hebrew. God's tongue, the rabbi had said. If you knew it, then you could talk to God. Who was He? He would learn about Him now—

The boy sitting nearest David, slid along the bench to his side. "Yuh jost stottin' cheder?"

"Yea."

227

"Uhh!" he groaned, indicating the rabbi with his eyes. "He's a louser! He hits!"

David regarded the rabbi with panicky eyes. He had seen boys slapped by teachers in school for disobedience, although he himself had never been struck. The thought of being flogged with that vicious scourge he had seen the rabbi produce sealed his lips. He even refused to answer when next the boy asked him whether he had any match-pictures to match, and hastily shook his head. With a shrug, the boy slid back along the bench to the place he had come from.

Presently, with the arrival of several late-comers, older boys, tongues once more began to wag and a hum of voices filled the room. When David saw that the rabbi brandished his scourge several times without wielding it, his fear abated somewhat. However, he did not venture to join in the conversation, but cautiously watched the rabbi.

The boy who had been reading when David had come in had finished, and his place was taken by a second who seemed less able to maintain the rapid drone of his predecessor. At first, when he faltered, the rabbi corrected him by uttering what was apparently the right sound, for the boy always repeated it. But gradually, as his pupil continued in his error, a harsh note of warning crept into the rabbi's voice. After awhile he began to yank the boy by the arm whenever he corrected him, then to slap him smartly on the thigh, and finally, just before the boy had finished, the rabbi cuffed him on the ear.

As time went by, David saw this procedure repeated in part or whole in the case of almost every other boy who read. There were several exceptions, and these, as far as David could observe, gained their exemption from punishment because the drone that issued from their lips was as breathless and uninterrupted as the roll of a drum. He also noticed that whenever the rabbi administered one of these manual corrections, he first dropped from his hand the little stick with which he seemed to set the pace on the page, and an instant later reached out or struck out, as the case might demand. So that, whenever he dropped the stick, whether to scratch his beard or adjust his skullcap or fish out a half-burned cigarette from a box, the pupil before him invariably jerked up an arm or ducked his head defensively. The dropping of that little stick, seemed to have become a warning to his pupils that a blow was on the way.

The light in the windows was waning to a blank pallor. The room was warm; the stagnant air had lulled even the most restive. Drowsily, David wondered when his turn would come.

"Aha!" he heard the rabbi sarcastically exclaim. "Is it you, Hershele, scholar from the land of scholars?"

This was addressed to the boy who had just slid into the vacant place before the book. David had observed him before, a fat boy with a dull face and an open mouth. By the cowed, sullen stoop of his shoulders, it was clear that he was not one in good standing with the rabbi.

"Herry is gonna loin," giggled one of the boys at David's side.

"Perhaps, today, you can glitter a little," suggested the rabbi with a freezing smile. "Who knows, a puppet may yet be made who can fart. Come!" He picked up the stick and pointed to the page.

The boy began to read. Though a big boy, as big as any that preceded him, he read more slowly and faltered more often than any of the others. It was evident that the rabbi was restraining his impatience, for instead of actually striking his pupil, he grimaced violently when he corrected him, groaned frequently, stamped his foot under the table and gnawed his under-lip. The other students had grown quiet and were listening. From their strained silence—their faces were by now half obscured in shadow— David was sure they were expecting some catastrophe any instant. The boy fumbled on. As far as David could tell, he seemed to be making the same error over and over again, for the rabbi kept repeating the same sound. At last, the rabbi's patience gave out. He dropped the pointer; the boy ducked, but not soon enough. The speeding plane of the rabbi's palm rang against his ear like a clapper on a gong.

"You plaster dunce!" he roared, "when will you learn a byse is a byse and not a vyse. Head of filth, where are your eyes?" He shook a menancing hand at the cringing boy and picked up the pointer.

But a few moments later, again the same error and again the same correction.

"May a demon fly off with your father's father! Won't blows help you? A byse, Esau, pig! A byse! Remember, a byse, even though you die of convulsions!"

The boy whimpered and went on. He had not uttered more than a few sounds, when again he paused on the awful brink, and as if out of sheer malice, again repeated his error. The last stroke of the bastinado! The effect on the rabbi was terrific. A frightful bellow clove his beard. In a moment he had fastened the pincers of his fingers on the cheeks of his howling pupil, and wrenching the boy's head from side to side roared out—

"A byse! A byse! A byse! All buttocks have only one eye. A byse! May your brains boil over! A byse! Creator of earth and firmament, ten thousand cheders are in this land and me you single out for torment! A byse! Most abject of God's fools! A byse!"

While he raved and dragged the boy's head from side to side with one hand, with the other he hammered the pointer with such fury against the table that David expected at any moment to see the slender stick buried in the wood. It snapped instead!

"He busted it!" gleefully announced the boy sitting near.

"He busted it!" the suppressed giggle went round.

Horrified himself by what he saw, David wondered what the rest could possibly be so amused about.

"I couldn't see," the boy at the table was blubbering. "I couldn't see! It's dark in here!"

"May your skull be dark!" the rabbi intoned in short frenzied yelps, "and your eyes be dark and your fate be of such dearth and darkness that you will call a poppy-seed the sun and a carraway the moon. Get up! Away! Or I'll empty my bitter heart upon you!"

Tears streaming down his cheeks, and wailing loudly, the boy slid off the bench and slunk away.

"Stay here till I give you leave to go," the rabbi called after him. "Wipe your muddy nose. Hurry, I say! If you could read as easily as your eyes can piss, you were a fine scholar indeed!"

The boy sat down, wiped his nose and eyes with his coat-sleeve and quieted to a suppressed snuffling.

230

Glancing at the window, the rabbi fished in his pockets, drew out a match and lit the low gas jet sticking out from the wall over head. While he watched the visibility of the open book on the table, he frugally shaved down the light to a haggard leaf. Then he seated himself again, unlocked a drawer in the table and drew out a fresh stick which looked exactly like the one he had just broken. David wondered whether the rabbi whittled a large supply of sticks for himself, knowing what would happen to them.

"Move back!" He waved the boy away who had reluctantly slipped into the place just vacated before the table. "David Schearl!" he called out, tempering the harshness of his voice. "Come here, my gold."

Quailing with fright, David drew near.

"Sit down, my child," he was still breathing hard with exertion. "Don't be alarmed." He drew out of his pocket a package of cigarette-papers and a tobacco pouch, carefully rolled a cigarette, took a few puffs, then snuffed it out and put it into an empty cigarette box. David's heart pounded with fear. "Now then," he turned the leaves of a book beside him to the last page. "Show me how blessed is your understanding." He drew David's tense shoulder down toward the table, and picking up the new stick, pointed to a large hieroglyph at the top of the page. "This is called Komitz. You see? Komitz. And this is an Aleph. Now, whenever one sees a Komitz under an Aleph, one says, Aw." His hot tobacco-laden breath swirled about David's face.

His mother's words about her rabbi flashed through his mind. He thrust them aside and riveted his gaze to the indicated letter as if he would seal it on his eyes.

"Say after me," continued the rabbi, "Komitz-Aleph—Aw!"

David repeated the sounds.

"So!" commanded the rabbi. "Once more! Komitz-Aleph-Aw!"

And after David had repeated it several times. "And this," continued the rabbi pointing to the next character "is called Bais, and a Komitz under a Bais—Baw! Say it! Komitz-Bais-Baw!"

"Komitz-Bais—Baw!" said David.

"Well done! Again."

And so the lesson progressed with repetition upon repetition. Whether out of fear or aptitude, David went through these first

231

steps with hardly a single error. And when he was dismissed, the rabbi pinched his cheek in praise and said:

"Go home. You have an iron head!"

"Odds!" said Izzy.

"Evens!" said Solly.

"Skinner!" said Izzy. "Don' hold back yuh fingers till yuh see wad I'm puttin' oud."

They were gambling for pointers as usual, and David stood by watching the turns of fortune. In other corners of the yard were others engrossed in the same game. There were a great many pointers in circulation to-day—someone had rifled the rabbi's drawer. Nothing else had been taken, neither his phylacteries, nor his clock, nor his stationery, nothing except his pointers. He had been furious, but since everyone else had looked blank, he hadn't been able to convict anyone. Yet here they were, all gambling for them. David was amused. In fact everything that had to do with pointers amused him. They were one of the few things that relieved the dullness of the cheder. He had thought when he first saw them that the rabbi whittled them out himself, but he soon found out he was wrong. The rabbi broke so many that that would have taken all day. No, the pointers were just ordinary lollipop sticks. And even that had been amusing. An incongruous picture had risen in his mind: He saw his severe, black-bearded rabbi wearing away an all-day sucker. But his fellow-pupils soon enlightened him. It was they who brought the rabbi the lollipop sticks. A gift of pointers meant a certain amount of leniency on the rabbi's part, a certain amount of preference. But the gift had to be substantial, else the rabbi forgot about it, and since few of his pupils could afford more than one lollipop a day, they gambled for them. Izzy's luck to-day was running high.

"Yuh god any more?" he asked.

"Yea," said Solly. "Make or break! Odds!"

"Waid a secon'. I'm all wet." He bent sideways and wrung his knee-pants and coattails. They had been arguing so violently a little while ago that someone in an adjacent house had thrown a bagful of water into their midst. Izzy had caught the brunt of it.

"Yowooee!" From a distance a long-drawn cat-call.

They looked around. "Who is it?"

"I'll see." Yonk who was standing near the fence shinnied up a washpole. "It's Moish," he announced. "He's t'ree fences."

"Only t'ree fences?" Contemptuously they resumed their game.

There was an approaching scuff and clatter. Moish climbed over the fence. "Any janitors?" he asked.

"No janitors," said Yonk patronizingly and slid down the wash-pole. "Yuh don' make enough noise, dat's why. Yuh oughta hea' Wildy."

"Who don' make enough noise? I hollered loud like anyt'ing. Who beats?"

"Who'djuh t'ink? Wildy beats. He god faw fences an' one jani-tor. Mrs. Lechtenstein on seven-sixty-eight house. She went smack wit' de broom, but Wildy ducked."

Fence-climbing was one of the ways by which the rabbi's pupils entered the cheder. The doorway that led into the cheder yard was too prosaic for most of them; they preferred to carve their own routes. And the champion of this, as of everything else, was Wildy. Wildy was nearing his thirteenth birthday and con-sequently his 'bar mitzvah,' which made him one of the oldest boys in the cheder. He was the idol of everyone and had even threatened to punch the rabbi in the nose.

"W'ea's Wildy now?" someone asked.

"He's waitin' fuh Shaih an' Toik t' comm down," Yonk looked significantly up at one of the houses. "He's gonna show em dey ain't de highest ones wad comms into de cheder."

"I god t'ree poinders," said Moish. "Who'll match me?"

"I'll play yuh." Izzy had just cleaned out his opponent. "W'ea didja ged 'em? From de swipe?"

"Naa. Dey's two goils in my class, an' anudder kid—a goy. So dey all bought lollipops, an' de goy too. So I follered dem aroun' an' aroun' an' den w'en dey finished, dey trowed away de sticks. So I picked 'em up. Goys is dumb."

"Lucky guy," they said enviously.

It took more than luck though, as David very well knew. It took a great deal of patience. He had tried that method of collect-ing lollipop sticks himself, but it had proved too tedious. Anyway he didn't really have to do it. He happened to be bright enough to avoid punishment, and could read Hebrew as fast as anyone, although he still didn't know what he read. Translation, which was called Chumish, would come later.

"Yowooee!" The cry came from overhead this time. They looked up. Shaih and Toik, the two brothers who lived on the third floor back had climbed out on their fire-escapes. They were the only ones in the cheder privileged to enter the yard via the fire-escape ladders—and they made the most of it. The rest watched enviously. But they had climbed down only a few steps, when again the cry, and now from a great height—

"Yowooee!"

Everyone gasped. It was Wildy and he was on the roof!

"I tol' yuh I wuz gonna comm down higher den dem!" With a triumphant shout he mounted the ladder and with many a flourish climbed down.

"Gee, Wildy!" they breathed reverently—all except the two brothers and they eyed him sullenly.

"We'll tell de janitor on you."

"I'll smack yuh one," he answered easily, and turning to the rest. "Yuh know wad I c'n do if one o' youz is game. I betcha I c'n go up on de fawt' flaw an' I betcha I c'n grab hol' from dat wash-line an' I betcha I c'n hol' id till sommbody pulls me across t' de wash-pole an I betcha I c'n comm down!"

"Gee, Wildy!"

"An' somm day I'm gonna stott way over on Avenyuh C an' jump all de fences in de whole two blocks!"

"Gee!"

"Hey, guys, I'm goin' in." Izzy had won the last of the pointers. "C'mon, I'm gonna give 'im."

"How many yuh god?" They trooped after him.

"Look!" There was a fat sheaf of them in his hand.

They approached the reading table. The rabbi looked up.

"I've got pointers for you, rabbi," said Izzy in Yiddish.

"Let me see them," was the suspicious answer. "Quite a contribution you're making."

Izzy was silent.

"Do you know my pointers were stolen yesterday?"

"Yes, I know."

"Well, where did you get these?"

"I won them."

"From whom?"

"From everybody."

"Thieves!" he shook his hand at them ominously. "Fortunately for you I don't recognize any of them."

Two months had passed since David entered the cheder. Spring had come and with the milder weather, a sense of wary contentment, a curious pause in himself as though he were waiting for some sign, some seal that would forever relieve him of watchfulness and forever insure his well-being. Sometimes he thought he had already beheld the sign—he went to cheder; he often went to the synagogue on Saturdays; he could utter God's syllables glibly. But he wasn't quite sure. Perhaps the sign would be revealed when he finally learned to translate Hebrew. At any rate, ever since he had begun attending cheder, life had leveled out miraculously, and this he attributed to his increasing nearness to God. He never thought about his father's job any longer. There was no more of that old dread of waiting for the cycle to fulfill itself. There no longer seemed to be any cycle. Nor did his mother ever appear to worry about his father's job; she too seemed reassured and at peace. And those curious secrets he had gleaned long ago from his mother's story seemed submerged within him and were met only at reminiscent street-corners among houses or in the brain. Everything unpleasant and past was like that, David decided, lost within one. All one had to do was to imagine that it wasn't there, just as the cellar in one's house could be conjured away if there were a bright yard between the hallway and the cellar-stairs. One needed only a bright yard. At times David almost believed he had found that brightness.

It was a few days before Passover. The morning had been so gay, warmer and brighter than any in the sheaf of Easter just past. Noon had been so full of promise—a leaf of Summer in the book of Spring. And all that afternoon he had waited, restless and inattentive, for the three o'clock gong to release him from school. Instead of blackboards, he had studied the sharp grids of

235

sunlight that brindled the red wall under the fire-escapes; and behind his tall geography book, had built a sail of a blotter and pencil to catch the mild breeze that curled in through the open window. Miss Steigman had caught him, had tightly puckered her lips (the heavy fuzz above them always darkened when she did that) and screamed:

"Get out of that seat, you little loafer! This minute! This very minute! And take that seat near the door and stay there! The audacity!" She always used that word, and David always wondered what it meant. Then she had begun to belch, which was what she always did after she had been made angry.

And even in his new seat, David had been unable to sit still, had fidgeted and waited, fingered the grain of his desk, stealthily rolled the sole of his shoe over a round lead pencil, attempted to tie a hair that had fallen on his book into little knots. He had waited and waited, but now that he was free, what good was it? The air was darkening, the naked wind was spinning itself a grey conch of the dust and rubbish scooped from the gutter. The street-cleaner was pulling on his black rain-coat. The weather had cheated him, that's all! He couldn't go anywhere now. He'd get wet. He might as well be the first one in the cheder. Disconsolately, he crossed the street.

But how did his mother know this morning it was going to rain? She had gone to the window and looked out, and then she said, the sun is up too early. Well what if it—Whee!

Before his feet a flat sheet of newspaper, driven by a gust of damp wind, whipped into the air and dipped and fluttered languidly, melting into sky. He watched it a moment and then quickened his step. Above store windows, awnings were heaving and bellying upward, rattling. Yelling, a boy raced across the gutter, his cap flying before him.

"Wow! Look!" The shout made him turn around.

"Shame! Shame! Everybody knows your name." A chorus of boys and girls chanted emphatically. "Shame! Shame! Everybody knows your name."

Red and giggling a big girl was thrusting down the billow of her dress. Above plump, knock-kneed legs, a glimpse of scalloped, white drawers. The wind relenting, the dress finally sank.

236

David turned round again, feeling a faint disgust, a wisp of the old horror. With what prompt spasms the mummified images in the brain started from their niches, aped former antics and lapsed. It recalled that time, way long ago. Knish and closet. Puh! And that time when two dogs were stuck together. Puh! Threw water that man. Shame! Shame!

"Sophe-e!" Above him the cry. "Sophe-e!"

"Ye-es, Mama-a!" from a girl across the street.

"Comm opstehs! Balt!"

"Awaa!"

"Balt or I'll give you! Nooo!"

With a rebellious shudder, the girl began crossing the street. The window slammed down.

Pushing a milk-stained, rancid baby carriage before them, squat buttocks waddled past, one arm from somewhere dragging two reeling children, each hooked by its hand to the other, each bouncing against the other and against their mother like tops, flagging and whipped. A boy ran in front of the carriage. It rammed him.

"Ow! Kencha see wea yuh goin?" He rubbed his ankle.

"Snott nuzz! Oll—balt a frosk, Oll—give!"

"Aaa! Buzjwa!"

A drop of rain spattered on his chin.

—It's gonna—

He flung his strap of books over his shoulder and broke into a quick trot.

—Before I get all wet.

Ahead of him, flying toward the shore beyond the East River, shaggy clouds trooped after their van. And across the river the white smoke of nearer stacks were flattened out and stormy as though the stacks were the funnels of a flying ship. In the gutter, wagon wheels trailed black ribbons. Curtains overhead paddled out of open windows. The air had shivered into a thousand shrill, splintered cries, wedged here and there by the sudden whoop of a boy or the impatient squawk of a mother. At the doorway to the cheder corridor, he stopped and cast one lingering glance up and down the street. The black sidewalks had cleared. Rain shook out wan tresses in the gathering dark. Against the piebald press of

237

cloud in the craggy furrow of the west, a lone flag on top of a school steeple blew out stiff as a key. In the shelter of a doorway, across the gutter, a cluster of children shouted in monotone up at the sky:

"Rain, rain, go away, come again some oddeh day. Rain, rain, go away, come again some oddeh day. Rain, rain—"

He'd better go in before the rest of the rabbi's pupils came. They'd get ahead of him otherwise. He turned and trudged through the dim battered corridor. The yard was gloomy. Wash-poles creaked and swayed, pulleys jangled. In a window over-head, a bulky, barearmed woman shrilled curses at someone behind her and hastily hauled in the bedding that straddled the sills like bulging sacks.

"And your guts be plucked!" her words rang out over the yard. "Couldn't you tell me it was raining?"

He dove through the rain, skidded over the broken flagstones and fell against the cheder door. As he stumbled in, the rabbi, who was lighting the gas-jet, looked around.

"A black year befall you!" he growled. "Why don't you come in like a man?"

Without answering, he sidled meekly over to the bench beside the wall and sat down. What did he yell at him for? He hadn't meant to burst in that way. Gee! The growing gas-light revealed another pupil in the room whom he hadn't noticed before. It was Mendel. His neck swathed in white bandages, sickly white under the bleary yellow flicker of gas, he sat before the reading table, head propped by elbows. Mendel was nearing his bar mitzvah but had never learned to read Chumish because he had entered the cheder at a rather late age. He was lucky, so every one said, because he had a carbuncle on the back of his neck which pre-vented him from attending school. And so all week long, he had arrived first at the cheder. David wondered if he dared sit down beside him. The rabbi looked angry. However, he decided to venture it and crawled quietly over the bench beside Mendel. The pungent reek of medicine pried his nostrils.

—Peeuh! It stinks!

He edged away. Dull-eyed, droopy-lipped, Mendel glanced down at him and then turned to watch the rabbi. The latter drew a large blue book from a heap on the shelf and then settled himself on his pillowed chair.

"Strange darkness," he said, squinting at the rain-chipped window. "A stormy Friday."

David shivered. Beguiled by the mildness of noon, he had left the house wearing only his thin blue jersey. Now, without a fire in the round-bellied stove and without other bodies to lend their warmth to the damp room, he felt cold.

"Now," said the rabbi stroking his beard, "this is the 'Haftorah' to Jethro—something you will read at your bar mitzvah, if you live that long." He wet his thumb and forefinger and began pinching the top of each page in such a way that the whole leaf seemed to wince from his hand and flip over as if fleeing of its own accord. David noted with surprise that unlike the rabbi's other books this one had as yet none of its corners lopped off. "It's the 'Sedrah' for that week," he continued, "and since you don't know any Chumish, I'll tell you what it means after you've read it." He picked up the pointer, but instead of pointing to the page suddenly lifted his hand.

In spite of himself, Mendel contracted.

"Ach!" come the rabbi's impatient grunt. "Why do you spring like a goat? Can I hit *you?*" And with the blunt end of the pointer, he probed his ear, his swarthy face painfully rippling about his bulbous nose into the margins of his beard and skullcap. He scraped the brown clot of wax against the table leg and pointed to the page. "Begin, Beshnos mos."

"Beshnos mos hamelech Uziyahu vaereh es adonoi," Mendel swung into the drone.

For want of anything better to do, David looked on, vying silently with Mendel. But the pace soon proved too fast for him —Mendel's swift sputter of gibberish tripped his own laggard lipping. He gave up the chase and gazed vacantly at the rain-chipped window. In a house across the darkened yard, lights had been lit and blurry figures moved before them. Rain strummed on the roof, and once or twice through the steady patter, a muffled rumble filtered down, as if a heavy object were being dragged across the floor above.

—Bed on wheels. Upstairs. (His thoughts rambled absently

239

between the confines of the drone of the voice and the drone of the rain.) Gee how it's raining. It won't stop. Even if he finishes, I can't go. If he read Chumish, could race him, could beat him I bet. But that's because he has to stop . . . Why do you have to read Chumish? No fun . . . First you read, Adonoi elahenoo ababab, and then you say, And Moses said you mustn't, and then you read some more ababab and then you say, mustn't eat in the traife butcher store. Don't like it any way. Big brown bags hang down from the hooks. Ham. And all kinds of grey wurst with like marbles in 'em. Peeuh! And chickens without feathers in boxes, and little bunnies in that store on First Avenue by the elevated. In a wooden cage with lettuce. And rocks, they eat too, on those stands. Rocks all colors. They bust 'em open with a knife and shake out ketchup on the snot inside. Yich! and long, black, skinny snakes. Peeuh! Goyim eat everything. . . .

"Veeshma es kol adonoi omair es mi eshlach." Mendel was reading swiftly this afternoon. The rabbi turned the page. Overhead that distant rumbling sound.

—Bed on wheels again . . . But how did Moses know? Who told him? God told him. Only eat kosher meat, that's how. Mustn't eat meat and then drink milk. Mama don't care except when Bertha was looking! How she used to holler on her because she mixed up the meat-knives with the milk-knives. It's a sin. . . . So God told him eat in your own meat markets . . . That time with mama in the chicken market when we went. Where all the chickens ran around—cuckacucka—when did I say? Cucka. Gee! Funny. Some place I said. And then the man with a knife went zing! Eee! Blood and wings. And threw him down. Even kosher meat when you see, you don't want to eat—

"Enough!" The rabbi tapped his pointer on the table.

Mendel stopped reading and slumped back with a puff of relief.

"Now I'll tell you a little of what you read, then what it means. Listen to me well that you may remember it. Beshnas mos hamelech." The two nails of his thumb and forefinger met. "In the year that King Uzziah died, Isaiah saw God. And God was sitting on his throne, high in heaven and in his temple—Understand?" He pointed upward.

Mendel nodded, grimacing as he eased the bandage round his neck.

—Gee! And he saw Him. Wonder where? (David, his interest aroused, was listening intently. This was something new.)

"Now!" resumed the rabbi. "Around Him stood the angels, God's blessed angels. How beautiful they were you yourself may imagine. And they cried: Kadosh! Kadosh! Kadosh—Holy! Holy! Holy! And the temple rang and quivered with the sound of their voices. So!" He paused, peering into Mendel's face. "Understand?"

"Yeh," said Mendel understandingly.

—And angels there were and he saw 'em. Wonder if—

"But when Isaiah saw the Almighty in his majesty and His terrible light—Woe me! he cried, What shall I do! I am lost!" The rabbi seized his skullcap and crumpled it. "I, common man, have seen the Almighty, I, unclean one have seen him! Behold, my lips are unclean and I live in a land unclean—for the Jews at that time were sinful—"

—Clean? Light? Wonder if—? Wish I could ask him why the Jews were dirty. What did they do? Better not! Get mad. Where? (Furtively, while the rabbi, still spoke David leaned over and stole a glance at the number of the page.) On sixty-eight. After, maybe, can ask. On page sixty-eight. That blue book—Gee! it's God.

"But just when Isaiah let out this cry—I am unclean—one of the angels flew to the altar and with tongs drew out a fiery coal. Understand? With tongs. And with that coal, down he flew to Isaiah and with that coal touched his lips—Here!" The rabbi's fingers stabbed the air. "You are clean! And the instant that coal touched Isaiah's lips, then he heard God's own voice say, Whom shall I send? Who will go for us? And Isaiah spoke and—"

But a sudden blast of voices out doors interrupted him. Running feet stamped across the yard. The door burst open. A squabbling tussling band stormed the doorway, jamming it. Scuffling, laughing boisterously, they shoved each other in, yanked each other out—

"Leggo!"

"Leggo me!"

"Yuh pushed me in id, yuh lousy stinkuh!"

"Next after Davy," one flew toward the reading table.

"Moishe flopped inna puddle!"

"Hey! Don' led 'im in!"

"Next after Sammy!" Another bolted after the first.

"I come—!"

"Shah!" grated the rabbi. "Be butchered, all of you! You hear me! Not one be spared!"

The babel sank to an undertone.

"And you there, be maimed forever, shut that door."

The milling about the doorway dissolved.

"Quick! may your life be closed with it."

Someone pulled the door after him.

"And now, sweet Sammy," his voice took on a venomous, wheedling tone. "*Nex* are you? I'll give you *nex*. In your belly it will *nex*. Out of there! Wriggle!"

Sammy hastily scrambled back over the bench.

"And you too," he waved David away. "Go sit down over there." And when David hung back. "Quick! Or—!"

David sprang from the bench.

"And quiet!" he rasped. "As if your tongues had rotted." And when complete silence had been established. "Now," he said, rising. "I'll give you something to do— Yitzchuck!"

"Waauh! I didn' do nottin'!" Yitzchuck raised a terrified whine.

"Who asked you to speak? Come here!"

"Wadda yuh wan' f'om me?" Yitzchuck prepared to blubber.

"Sit here." He beckoned to the end of the bench which was nearest the reading table. "And don't speak to me in goyish. Out of there, you! And you, David, sit where you are— Simke!"

"Yea."

"Beside him. Srool! Moishe! Avrum! Yankel! Schulim!" He was gathering all the younger students into a group. "Schmiel! And you Meyer, sit here." With a warning glance, he went over to the closet behind his chair and drew out a number of small books.

"Aaa! Phuh!" Yitzchuck spat out in a whisper. "De lousy Hagaddah again!"

They sat silent until the rabbi returned and distributed the books. Moishe, seated a short distance away from David dropped his, but then pounced upon it hastily, and for the rabbi's benefit, kissed it and looked about with an expression of idiotic piety.

"First, louse-heads," began the rabbi when he had done distributing the books, "the Four Questions of the Passover. Read them again and again. But this time let them flow from your lips like a torrent. And woe to that plaster dunce who still cannot say them in Yiddish! Blows will he scoop like sand! And when you have done that, turn the leaves to the 'Chad Godya.' Read it over. But remember, quiet as death— Well?" Shmaike had raised his hand as though he were in school. "What do you want?"

"Can't we hear each other?"

"Mouldered brains! Do you still need to hear each other? Do then. But take care I don't hear a goyish word out of you." He went back to his chair and sat down. For a few seconds longer his fierce gaze raked the long bench, then his eyes dropped momentarily to the book before him. "I was telling you," he addressed Mendel, "how Isaiah came to see God and what happened after—"

But as if his own words had unleashed theirs, a seething of whispers began to chafe the room.

"You hea' me say it. You hea' me! Shid on you. C'mon Solly, you hea' me. Yuh did push! Mendy's god a bendige yet on—"

"Said whom shall I send?" The rabbi's words were baffling on thickening briers of sound. "Who will go for us?"

"Izzy Pissy! Cock-eye Mulligan! Mah nishtanah halilaw hazeh — Wanna play me Yonk?"

—Couldn't ask him though (David's eyes merely rested on the page). Get mad. Maybe later when I have to read. Where was it? Yea. Page sixty-eight. I'll say, on page sixty-eight in that blue book that's new, where Mendel read, you were saying that man saw God. And a light—

"How many? I god more den you. Shebchol haleylos onu achlim— I had a mockee on mine head too. Wuz you unner de awningh? Us all wuz. In de rain."

"And tell this people, this fallen people—"

"Yea, and I'll kickyuh innee ass! Odds! Halaylaw hazeh kulo mazo—So from t'rowin' sand on my head I god a big mockee. I seen a blitz just w'en I commed in."

—Where did he go to see Him? God? Didn't say. Wonder if the rabbi knows? Wish I could ask. Page sixty-eight. Way, way, way, maybe. Where? Gee! Some place, me too . . . When I— When I—in the street far away . . . Hello, Mr. Highwood, good-bye Mr. Highwood. Heee! Funny!

"C'mere Joey, here's room. De rebbeh wants—Fences is all slippery. Now wadda yuh cry?"

"Nor ever be healed, nor ever clean."

"A blitz, yuh dope! Hey Solly, he says—Shebchol haleylos onu ochlim—Yea, my fadder'll beat chaw big brudder. Evens!"

—Some place Isaiah saw Him, just like that. I bet! He was sitting on a chair. So he's got chairs, so he can sit. Gee! Sit Shit! Sh! Please God, I didn't mean it! Please God, somebody else said it! Please—

"So hoddy you say blitz wise guy? Moishee loozed his bean shooduh! And den after de sand I pud wawduh on duh head, so—Lousy bestid! Miss Ryan tooked it!"

"How long? I asked. Lord, how long—"

—And why did the angel do it? Why did he want to burn Isaiah's mouth with coal? He said, You're clean. But coal makes smoke and ashes. So how clean? Couldn't he just say, Your mouth is clean? Couldn't he? Why wasn't it clean, anyway? He didn't wash it, I bet. So that . . .

"A lighten', yuh dope. A blitz! Kent'cha tuck Englitch? Ha! Ha! Sheor yerokos halaylo hazeh—Dat's two on dot! I wuz shootin chalk wid it. Somm bean shooduh! My fodder'll give your fodder soch a kick—"

—With a zwank, he said it was. Zwank. Where did I see? Zwank some place. Mama? No. Like in blacksmith shop by the river. Pincers and horseshoe. Yes must be. With pincers, zwank means pincers. So why with pincers? Coal was hot. That's why. But he was a angel. Is angels afraid? Afraid to get burned? Gee! Must have been hot, real hot. How I jumped when the rabbi pushed out with his fingers when he said coal. Nearly thought it was me. Wonder if Isaiah hollered when the coal touched him. Maybe angel-coal don't burn live people. Wonder—

"Dere! Chinky shows! Id's mine! How many fences didja go? I tore it f'om a tree in duh pock, mine bean-shooduh! T'ree fences. So a lighten den, wise guy!"

"And the whole land waste and empty."

"T'ree is a lie, mine fodder says. Yea? Matbilim afilu pa'am echos halaylo hazeh—Always wear yuh hat when a lighten' gives—"

—He said dirty words, I bet. Shit, pee, fuckenbestit—Stop! You're sayin' it yourself. It's a sin again! That's why he—Gee! I didn't mean it. But your mouth don't get dirty. I don't feel no dirt. (He rolled his tongue about.) Maybe inside. Way, way in, where you can't taste it. What did Isaiah say that made his mouth dirty? Real dirty, so he'd know it was? Maybe—

"Shebchol haleleylos onu ochlim— De rain wedded my cocka-mamy! Ow! Leggo! Yuh can't cover books wit' newspaper. My teacher don' let. An aftuh she took mine been-shooduh, she pinched me by duh teet! Lousy bestid! Bein yoshvim uvein mesubim. So wad's de nex' woid? Mine hen'ball went down duh sewuh! Now, I god six poinduhs!"

—You couldn't do it with a regular coal. You'd burn all up. Even hot tea if you drink—ooh! But where could you get angel-coal? Mr. Ice-man, give me a pail of angel-coal. Hee! Hee! In a cellar is coal. But other kind, black coal, not angel coal. Only God had angel-coal. Where is God's cellar I wonder? How light it must be there. Wouldn't be scared like I once was in Brownsville. Remember?

"C'mon chick! Hey Louie! Yuh last! Wed mine feed! Look! Me! Yea! Hea! Two!"

—Angel-coal. In God's cellar is—

All the belated ones had straggled in. A hail of jabbering now rocked the cheder.

"And-not-a-tree—" As the rabbi stooped lower and lower, his voice shot up a steep ladder of menace. "Shall-be-upright in the land!" He straightened, scaling crescendo with a roar. "Noo!" His final shattering bellow mowed down the last shrill reeds of voices. "Now it's my turn!" Smiling fiercely he rose, cat-o-nine in hand, and advanced toward the silent, cowering row. "Here!" the scourge whistled down, whacked against a thigh. "Here's for you!"

"Wow!"

"And you!"

"Ouch! Waddid I—do?"

"And you for your squirming tongue!"

"Leggo! Ooh!"

"And you that your rump is on fire! Now sit still!"

"Umph! Ow!"

"And you for your grin! And you for your nickering, and you for your bickering. Catch! Catch! Hold! Dance!"

The straps flew, legs plunged. Shrill squibs of pain popped up and down the bench. No one escaped, not even David. Wearied at length, and snorting for breath, the rabbi stopped and glared at them. Suppressed curses, whimpers, sniffles soughed from one end of the bench to the other.

"Shah!"

Even these died out.

"Now! To your books! Dig your eyes into them. The Four Questions. Noo! Begin! Ma nishtanaw."

"Mah nishtanaw halilaw hazeh," they bellowed, "mikawl halaylos. Sheb chol halaylos onu ochlim chametz umazoh."

"Schulim!" The rabbi's chin went down, his voice diving past it to an ominous bass. "Dumb are you?"

"Haliylaw hazeh." A new voice vigorously swelled the already lusty chorus, "kulo mazoh!"

When they had finished the four questions, repeated them and rendered them thrice into Yiddish—

"Now the chad godyaw," commanded the rabbi. "And with one voice. Hurry!"

Hastily, they turned the pages.

"Chad godyaw, chad godyaw," they bayed raggedly, "disabin abaw bis rai zuzaw, chad godyaw, chad godyaw—"

"Your teeth fall out, Simkeh," snarled the rabbi, grinning venomously, "what are you laughing at?"

"Nuttin!" protested Simkeh in an abused voice. "I wasn't laughing!" He was though—some one had been chanting "fot God Yaw" instead of Chad-Godyaw.

"So!" said the rabbi sourly when they had finished. "And now where is the blessed understanding that remembers yesterday? Who can render this into Yiddish? Ha? Where?"

A few faltering ones raised their hands.

"But all of it!" he warned. "Not piece-meal, all of it without stuttering. Or—" He snapped the cat-o'-nine. "The noodles!"

Scared, the volunteers lowered their hands.

"What? None? Not a single one." His eyes swept back and forth. "Oh, you!" With a sarcastic wave of the hand, he flung back the offers of the older, Chumish students. "It's time you mastered this feat! No one!" He wagged his head at them bitterly. "May you never know where your teeth are! Hi! Hi! none strives to be a Jew any more. Woe unto you! Even a goy knows more about his filth than you know of holiness. Woe! Woe!" He glared at David accusingly. "You too? Is your head full of turds like the rest of them? Speak!"

"I know it," he confessed, but at the same time feigned sullenness lest he stir the hatred of the others.

"Well! Have you ribs in your tongue? Begin! I'm waiting!"

"One kid, one only kid," cautiously he picked up the thread, "one kid that my father bought for two zuzim. One kid, one only kid. And a cat came and ate the kid that my father had bought for two zuzim. One kid, one only kid. And a dog came and bit the cat that ate the kid that my father bought for two zuzim. One kid, one only kid." He felt more and more as he went on as if the others were crouching to pounce upon him should he miss one rung in the long ladder of guilt and requital. Carefully, he climbed past the cow and the butcher and the angel of death. "And then the Almighty, blessed be He— (*Gee! Last. Nobody after. Didn't know before. But sometime, Mama, Gee!*) Unbidden, the alien thoughts crowded into the gap. For an instant he faltered. (No! No! Don't stop!) "Blessed be He," he repeated hurriedly, "killed the angel of death, who killed the butcher, who killed the ox, who drank the water, that quenched the fire, that burned the stick, that beat the dog, that bit the cat, that ate the kid, that my father bought for two zuzim. One kid, one only kid!" Breathlessly he came to an end, wondering if the rabbi were angry with him for having halted in the middle.

But the rabbi was smiling. "So!" he patted his big palms to-

gether. "This one I call my child. This is memory. This is intellect. You may be a great rabbi yet—who knows!" He stroked his
black beard with a satisfied air and regarded David a moment,
then suddenly he reached his hand into his pocket and drew out a
battered black purse.

A murmur of incredulous astonishment rose from the bench.

Snapping open the pronged, metal catch, the rabbi jingled the
coins inside and pinched out a copper. "Here! Because you have
a true Yiddish head. Take it!"

Automatically, David lifted his hand and closed it round the
penny. The rest gaped silently.

"Now come and read," he was peremptory again. "And the
rest of you dullards, take care! Let me hear you wink and I'll tear
you not into shreds, but into shreds of shreds!"

A little dazed by the windfall, David followed him to the reading bench and sat down. While the rabbi carefully rolled himself
a cigarette, David gazed out of the window. The rain had
stopped, though the yard was still dark. He could sense a strange
quietness holding the outdoors in its grip. Behind him, the first
whisper flickered up somewhere along the bench. The rabbi lit his
cigarette, shut the book from which Mendel had been reading and
pushed it to one side.

—Could ask him now, I bet. He gave me a penny. About
Isaiah and the coal. Where? Yes. Page sixty-eight. I could ask—

Chaa! Wuuh! Thin smoke glanced off the table. The rabbi
reached over for the battered book and picked up the pointer.

"Rabbi?"

"Noo?" He pinched over the leaves.

"When Mendel was reading about that—that man who you
said, who—" He never finished. Twice through the yard, as
though a lantern had been swung back and forth above the rooftops, violet light rocked the opposite walls—and darkness for a
moment and a clap of thunder and a rumbling like a barrel
rolling down cellar stairs.

"Shma yisroel!" the rabbi ducked his head and clutched
David's arm. "Woe is me!"

"Ow!" David squealed. And the pressure on his arm relaxing,
giggled.

Behind him the sharp, excited voices. "Yuh seen it! Bang! Bang wot a bust it gave! I tol' yuh I seen a blitz before!"

"Shah!" The rabbi regained his composure. "Lightning before the Passover! A warm summer." And to David as if remembering, "Why did you cry out and why did you laugh?"

"You pinched me," he explained cautiously, "and then—"

"Well?"

"And then you bent down—like us when you drop the pointer, and then I thought—"

"Before God," the rabbi interrupted, "none may stand upright."

—Before God.

"But what did you think?"

"I thought it was a bed before. Upstairs. But it wasn't."

"A bed! It wasn't!" He stared at David. "Don't play the fool with me because I gave you a penny." He thrust the book before him. "Come then!" he said brusquely. "It grows late."

—Can't ask now.

"Begin! Shohain ad mawrom—"

"Shohain ad mawrom vekawdosh shmo vakawsuv ronnu zadekim ladonoi." Thought lapsed into monotone.

After a short reading, the rabbi excused him, and David slid off the bench and went over to where the rest were sitting to get his strap of books. Schloime, who held them in his lap, had risen with alacrity as he approached and proffered them to him.

"Dey wanted t' take dem, but I was holdin' 'em." He informed him. "Watcha gonna buy?"

"Nuttin."

"Aa!" And eagerly. "I know w'ea dere's orange-balls—eight fuh a cent."

"I ain' gonna ged nuttin."

"Yuh stingy louse!"

The others had swarmed about. "I told yuh, yuh wouldn' get nuttin for holdin' his books. Yaah, yuh see! Aaa, let's see duh penny. We'll go witchah. Who couldn'a said dat!"

"Shah!"

They scattered back to the bench. David eased his way through the door.

LILLIAN WALD

Lillian Wald was born in Cincinnati, Ohio, on March 10, 1867, the daughter of Max and Minnie (Schwarz) Wald. She graduated from the Training School for Nurses at New York Hospital and became a registered nurse. This apparently remained her proudest boast during a life in which so many honors came to her. She also attended the Women's Medical College in New York City.

In 1893, she founded the Henry Street Settlement with which her name has been associated ever since. The list of her public services is long. Among the more important posts that she occupied were those on the New York State Board of Immigration, the National and New York Child Labor Committees, the American League to Abolish Capital Punishment, the New York Urban League, and the Women's International League for Peace and Freedom.

In addition to *Windows on Henry Street,* from which an excerpt appears here, she wrote *The House on Henry Street* and articles on "nursing, social subjects, human betterment." She was a lecturer at various times at Teachers College and at the New York School of Social Work. She served as a member of President Wilson's Industrial Council and participated in President Hoover's White House Conference on Health and Protection. She is credited with originating the idea of a Federal Children's Bureau.

She received honorary LL.D. degrees from Mount Holyoke College in 1912 and from Smith College in 1930. She also received gold medals from the National Institute of the Social Sciences and from the Rotary Clubs of America in recognition of her lifelong services as sociologist, organizer, and publicist. The Henry Street Settlement, which she founded, eventually grew to a great size and attracted world-wide interest. She died in 1940.

Windows on Henry Street

From the dawn of time, children have touched the compassion, the imagination, the protective sense of people, but it is only recently that educators have recognized that adults too have a claim to further development. It is frequently argued that they should not be suffered to remain in a rut, that they should keep pace, at least to some extent, with their often arrogant youngsters. And also there is recognition among all people whose minds are not sealed that with the shortened days and weeks of work the use of increased unemployed time is most important. It is surprisingly easy for men and women who work hard, and who might think that with marriage and parenthood their part in life has been played, to be stirred to consciousness of their value as citizens and as individuals. Settlements have always tried to bring the generations together, as they have tried to bring races and nationalities together, and it has at times required no little manœuvering to awaken the children to pride in their "un-American" parents and to recognition of the gifts they have bestowed. This problem has been much discussed, and it now gains greater significance from the physical fact that there are more older people in the world than there were, that the expectation of life has increased ten years since 1900, and that with greater leisure there is possible a vital contribution on the part of the increased adult population.

On the Feast of Tabernacles in our Jewish neighborhood we set up on our roof a *sukkah* or booth, according to the ritual prescribed in Leviticus for this festival of the "ingathering." The

Selection from Lillian Wald's *Windows on Henry Street*, published by Little Brown, Boston, 1934.

253

proudest participant in the service is an old man from a neighborhood tenement who chants the religious songs inspired for the
occasion hundreds—perhaps thousands—of years ago. The admiration felt for him filters down to the smart young people of
the clubs who are invited to the roof; and, after our demonstration of respect for old customs, the neighborhood takes part,
bringing fruits and cakes and homemade wine, according to tradition. There is no sense of intrusion, but rather of hospitality,
when guests who happen to be at the Settlement, though they
know little of Jewish customs, join in the celebration and are
moved by the beauty of this ceremony transferred from the
Orient to New York's East Side.

Changes in this observance symbolize the changes in the economic condition of the neighborhood. When I first came to the
East Side, I would see the pitiful, newly arrived immigrants
bargaining with the pushcart dealers for *lulab* (sprays of willow
or myrtle) and *esrog* (lemons), the greens and fruit traditionally
associated with the festival. Having no place to build the ceremonial booth, as their forebears did, they would lay branches
over the roof of the outdoor toilet, which bore a remote suggestion of the traditional *sukkah*. None of to-day's children know of
this sorry makeshift, and their reintroduction to the old customs
of the festival comes from people who see the spiritual message
and who love to have the beautiful preserved as an inheritance.

When the settlements wish to give an exhibition of ancient and
modern art they can draw upon their neighbors for beautiful old
bits. Lace, embroidery, pottery, carvings, jewelry, are treasured
as reminders of the old home. The young people are only now
beginning to appreciate these heirlooms. "Hundred per cent
Americanism" had led to a contemptuous feeling even toward
these. Some of the treasures given to me long ago by immigrants
I have now passed over to their grandchildren. In truth, I cannot
say that they always value them as I did.

The beautiful brasses and coppers that have delighted the
hearts of many collectors and made Allen Street famous have
been given away with great liberality. But few know that the
seven-branched candlestick that stands on so many non-Jewish
tables symbolizes the seven planets and the Sabbath prayer
through which God unites all.

Hospitality is a tradition in our neighborhood. One of the invitations most prized at Henry Street is that which bids us welcome to a Passover service. Despite the influences of liberalism within the faith, and scorn on the part of some of those who have broken with old traditions, it remains an impressive and a lovely ceremonial. So generous are the homes, even those with the fewest dollars, that homemade wine, an essential part of the Passover observance, is pressed upon acquaintances who are not of the faith, and sometimes unwisely. Our colored janitor once came to my door obviously under the influence of liquor. When I ventured to reprove him he said, speaking in the accents of one who has drunk too deeply, "Don' you worry—ish all ri'—ish holy Jewish wine."

Our neighbors share their old-country customs and skills not only with the Settlement but with one another. At a woman's club composed of different nationalities, an Italian housewife brought to the meeting a fragrant dish of spaghetti to show how the popular dish of her homeland should be cooked and eaten. This inspired a Russian Jewess to bring her *gefüllter Fisch*, most difficult to prepare and highly esteemed by true believers.

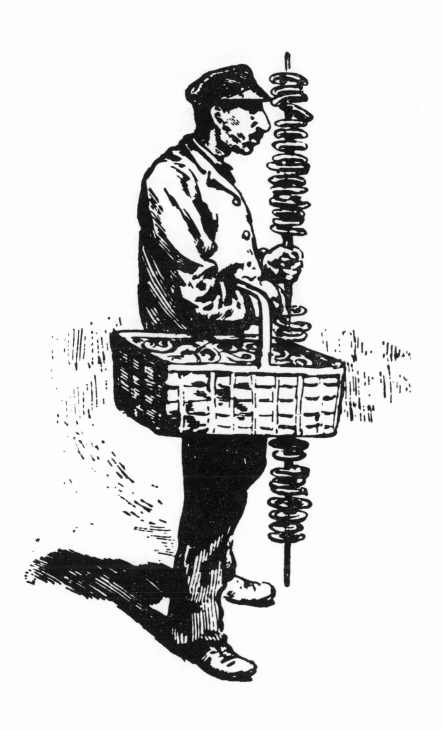

MARY KINGSBURY
SIMKHOVITCH

The founder and director of Greenwich House in New York, one of the best known of the settlement houses, which was started in 1902, was born in Newton, Massachusetts, September 8, 1867. She was the daughter of Colonel Isaac Franklin and Laura Davis (Holmes) Kingsbury. In 1899, she married Vladimir G. Simkhovitch, an economics professor at Columbia University.

She had received her B.S. degree from Boston University in 1890 and also attended for a time Radcliffe College, the University of Berlin, and Columbia University. She was a member of Phi Beta Kappa. She listed herself a member of the Episcopal Church and declared herself a Democrat in politics. Mayor La Guardia appointed her a member of the New York City Housing Authority and Governor Franklin D. Roosevelt appointed her to the New York State Board of Social Welfare. She was a member of the National Urban League and of the National Public Housing Conference. In addition to *Neighborhood*, from which we have taken an excerpt, she was the author of *City Worker's World* and of various articles in periodicals.

Neighborhood

Ashot rang out on the first night I spent at the College Settlement on Rivington Street. I put my head out the window. Allen Street, the heart of the red-light district, suddenly became silent. Then cries, and the rapid run of police. It was not a reassuring night and I felt shaken the next day. I marveled at the calm of Dr. Robbins, whose apprentice I was at the time, as we met for breakfast. But soon I settled like a submarine into the life of the neighborhood.

Rivington Street was crowded and noisy and rank with the smell of overripe fruit, hot bread and sweat-soaked clothing. The sun poured down relentlessly and welded the East Side together in one impress of fetid fertility. Neither in Phillips Street among my colored friends in Boston nor in the East End of London was there the vivid sense of a new and overpowering vitality such as emanated from the neighborhood of the College Settlement.

The settlement house itself was a beautiful old dwelling with heavy mahogany doors separating the two large rooms on the main floor. There was a spacious back yard bordered by homes of ranging sizes, some wooden, some brick. The yard was fitted up as a playground—one of the first in New York. Opposite the house was a wooden tenement. The basement of the house was the domain of Sarah, the cook, whose friendly understanding did much to endear the house to the neighborhood. In the front basement Miss Emily Wagner began the music school. It is said that one child practiced on one end of the piano and another on the other end. At any rate, violin lessons soon overflowed into the

Selection from Mary Kingsbury Simkhovitch's *Neighborhood*, published by W. W. Norton Company, New York, 1938.

basement hall. To Sarah's patience as well as to Miss Wagner's genius is due the immediate success of the music lessons. The neighborhood avidly responded to the opportunity; before my year was up a floor was engaged in the wooden house opposite, and the music school began to live its own life. Later it combined with the University Settlement Music School and then emerged into the Third Street Music School Settlement with a house of its own. The front room of the house was a library and assembly room. The back room, the residents' dining room, was used for clubs, or, together with the front room, for dancing, parties and meetings of all sorts.

As soon as I knew I was to be at the College Settlement, I read Emil Franzos and the stories of A. Cahan to try to familiarize myself with the background of the newcomers in the district, who were largely from little Jewish towns in Rumania, Galicia, Russia and Poland. The language was a difficulty, but German helped greatly. Of course I took Yiddish lessons. My teacher was a club boy at the University Settlement, now a well-known educator. Soon I could decipher all signs haltingly, read the Yiddish newspapers and enjoy the Yiddish theater. Life in the East Side at that time was far more picturesque than now. The Yiddish drama was good before it was "Americanized." The motion-picture house had not appeared. There were good literary clubs, and I availed myself of every opportunity to meet leaders of local opinion. In the evening at ten o'clock, when clubs and evening events at the Settlement disbanded, many of us would meet for tea at Lorber's on Grand Street to discuss East Side matters and talk over the excitements of the day. For each day we discovered something new: some teacher's difficulties in a near-by school, some boy arrested and taken to court, some girl abandoned by her family.

There was no Seward Park in those days. But the Outdoor Recreation League used to meet at the Settlement, and Dr. Robbins, the head worker, brought me in touch with the embryonic movement for public playgrounds. Mr. Charles Stover and Mr. James Paulding of the University Settlement were the leading local spirits in this association. Finally, Seward Park was secured and the playground idea visualized.

When, after my apprenticeship of a few months, I took charge of the house, I was prepared for the responsibility in one way only: by my intense interest in and admiration for the East Side. My own special task was the Sunday Evening Economics Club I formed that winter. Many of the members of the Club were more deeply versed than I in economic literature. Not accustomed to debate, I left that to the Club. My task was rather to open the minds of the members to another outlook than their own, just as their service to me was to introduce me to the intensity, the conviction, the aggressive thought of the Jewish mind. We got along famously, and friendships formed then have never been broken.

What happened seldom in London is a commonplace here. Today the members of that Club, who then lived in direst poverty in crowded rooms of the old "dumbbell" unimproved tenements, are now living on Riverside Drive and call for me in their motors to visit them. "Up from Slavery" was not Booker T. Washington's monopoly. From the slavery of the tenement sweatshop have arisen leaders in industry, in education, in art and in political life. Indeed, the old East Side was the fertile producer of today's judges, teachers, actors, musicians, playwrights and leaders of New York. I remember writing a little pamphlet at that time on East Side socialism and what it really signified to its adherents. For the real university of the East Side was Marx's *Capital*. Read like the Bible with faith, like the Bible it formed the taste and molded the life of its readers. Socialism as an economic theory is one thing; as an education it is another. It is what we are excited about that educates us. What the East Side was excited about was socialism. The press, the clubs, the theater, all were centered in the thought of a changed order. The Broadway of the garment industry had only begun its materialistic inroads. America knew little of foreign dogma and paid no attention to the convictions of immigrants. The Populist party in the West and the Knights of Labor had attempted to unite all of labor into one living force— and these were the only outstanding movements that had disturbed the serenity of the country in its triumphal march toward industrial supremacy. The country took no pains to present to the East Side the opportunities open in the West. The life of the

West, the village, the forest, the great riverways, the yeasty give-and-take of American life gradually developing a common consciousness and civilization were unknown to the old East Side. No effort was made to bring together such differing outlooks.

The Jewish mind is centripetal; everything it discovers it appropriates, and in that way becomes richer and more fertile, like an old garden plot well cultivated. But it appropriates only what comes within its grasp. And America felt little responsibility for offering to its newcomers all its possibilities.

The Yiddish newspapers, the Yiddish theater, Yiddish society as a whole, presented a picture of far greater concentration than at present. The East Side was not "Americanized" as it is today. In 1898 the Bowery was in its full flower and flavor of stage-villainy. Bread lines, missions, shooting galleries and shops where black eyes and bruises could be artistically touched up to resemble nature in its pristine innocence, gave a tang to the old Bowery long since mellowed, decayed and innocuous. Precious were the days of Big Tim Sullivan, who drew tribute from a whole region. His large picnics and outings, his crowded clubrooms, his ability to keep a crowd of henchmen together, his sense of the group and his knowledge of what could be accomplished through political organization based on meeting ordinary social needs, made of him a truly notable figure. Among lesser lights of the time was Martin Engel, leader of the Eighth Ward. At election time he used to drive through our ward in an open barouche, his fingers laden with diamonds, and more diamonds shone from his cravat. The intellectual Jewish East Side for the most part did not comprehend the game played by the political leaders. But they dimly realized what benefits accrued from keeping in with the forceful ones.

Jewish leadership was largely confined to the socialist party or parties, for that was the time when the socialist Labor party and the Social Democratic party were at swords' points. The socialist groups were passionately interested in theories, the Bowery's politicians in profit. There was little interest in a more realistic political program. Occasionally the conditions of work in the tobacco trade or the garment industry would become a matter of public concern, but political campaigns would overlook the real issues of East Side life.

As the political morale of the city sank, a reaction necessarily set in and the "good government club" era opened. The object of these clubs was to replace "bad" government by "good." It was a valuable but negative period. It had, not a social program, but the very natural desire to "drive the rascals out." To attack an evil is a simple political project. It has the merit of combining elements which fly apart when a constructive program is called for. The political attack, like a military offensive, places the opposition in a position of defense, which is always psychologically weak. But there is this difference between the political attack and the military offensive: the latter has an objective and the former is often a colorless effort with no appeal to the profounder instincts of man. "Turn 'em out" wears very thin after a while, when it is seen that the political and social structure remains much as it was before "goodness" came in. Political strength depends either on dramatic issues easily understood, or upon sound organization. Dramatic issues are few but can be readily grasped by the voters as a whole. Crime waves, the police, graft —these issues last well, even though threadbare. But in organization the reform groups are often inferior. They lose interest between campaigns; they go to the country when primaries approach. There is all the difference in the world between those who favor a policy and those who have a stake in it.

The first Seth Low campaign was fought during my year at the College Settlement. In local halls congregations of pious Jews saying their Shabbos Eve prayers folded their shawls and were supplanted by feverish political meetings. A clergyman in a neighborhood mission had told of the horrors of the Allen Street district. Bishop Potter had championed his witness. The hat was in the ring. Though victory that year was but temporary, it marked a real change in public opinion. After each serious and successful attempt to place government on a higher basis than profit for the benefited, the political life of the city has registered a permanent advance. There is graft and immorality in New York, but the old red-light days have gone.

The old German residents of the East Side rapidly moved

north and were replaced by a mass of Jewish immigrants fleeing from persecution. Little old ramshackle wooden houses were pulled down and in their place arose the double-decker "dumb-bell" tenements. This type of dwelling once won a prize in a contest for suitable dwellings for the poor. Its financial rewards were so great that it soon became the dominant type in New York. The twenty-four-family house came to stay. Through the air shafts (or small interior courts) vermin made their way, and at the bottom garbage and refuse collected. Privacy was rendered impossible. Soiling sights and sounds became a part of children's lives.

ANZIA YEZIERSKA

Anzia Yezierska was born in Poland when it was part of the Russian Empire in 1885, the daughter of Bernard and Pearl Yezierska. She came to this country in 1901 and was largely self-educated. She knew from first-hand experience the factories and sweatshops which later entered into her stories. She also served as a cook for private families.

She began to write stories about East Side life in 1918, and in 1919 she was the author of a long story, "Fat of the Land," which Edward J. O'Brien, the well-known anthologist of that day, chose as the best story published that year in the United States. It was a story which resembled in some respects (of plot and character, though not in the acridness of the tone in which it was told) the better-known story by Thyra Samter Winslow on the same subject (the disillusionments inseparable from the economic and social climbing of the immigrant Jews), which she called "A Cycle of Manhattan" and which has become part of many collections of American stories.

In 1920, a group of her stories was collected and published under the title *Hungry Hearts*. For some unlikely reason, this won the attention of Hollywood and was made into a not very successful motion picture in 1922. The difference that this made in her way of living is the subject of the section of her autobiography chosen for inclusion in this anthology. The autobiography itself was published in 1950 under the title *Red Ribbon on a White Horse*, with an Introduction by the poet W. H. Auden. Others of her books include *Salomé of the Tenements* (1922), *Children of Loneliness* (1923), *Bread Givers* (1925), *Arrogant Beggar* (1927), and *All I Could Never Be* (1932).

Twentieth Century Authors, in its entry on her, says: "Miss Yezierska was a vocal and belligerent immigrant writer, less meek and receptive than Mary Antin." It quotes a review of Carl Van Doren's of *Hungry Hearts* in which he said: "When she leaves the East Side neighborhood in which her art is native, she never quite has the look of reality." And Lyman Bryson, writing in the *New York Times* concerning her autobiography, *Red Ribbon on a White Horse,* noted that "the fierceness of temperament that has made life so hard for her shows in her writing, which is nervous, direct, and passionate. . . . She tells the disturbing truth about her own soul."

In her book *Children of Loneliness,* she has said: "Writing is to me a confession—not a profession. I know a man, a literary hack, who calls himself a dealer in words. He can write to order on any subject he is hired to write about. I often marvel at the ease with which he can turn from literary criticism to politics to psychoanalysis. A fatal fluency enables him to turn out thousands of words a day in the busy factory of his brain, without putting anything of himself into it." But if this method of composition lent her strength, it was also an important source of weakness and explains why she ran dry of inspiration periodically.

Her most important message to the world had been stated in *Hungry Hearts* when she wrote in an oft-quoted passage: "Until America can release the heart as well as train the hand of the immigrant, he would forever remain driven back upon himself, corroded by the very richness of the unused gifts in his soul." To Mary Antin, America had been a release to the heart from the very moment she landed in this country and possibly even before; Miss Yezierska proved to be one of those harder to please. Yet her demands do not seem in retrospect to have been excessive. In fact, her insistence that the immigrant needed something more than mere technical training (to set him up in a trade or be capable of seizing an opportunity to start a business) seems entirely salutary. To one of her teachers in a school for immigrants, who had attempted to channel her bursting energies along conventional, utilitarian lines, she had once said boldly: "Ain't thoughts useful? Does America want only the work from my body, my hands? Ain't it thoughts that turn over the world? . . .

Us immigrants want to be people—not 'hands'—not slaves of the belly! And it's the chance to think that makes people. . . . I came to give out all the fine things that were choked in me in Russia. I came to help America to make a new world. . . . They said, in America I could open my heart and fly free in the air—to sing— to dance—to live—to love. . . . Here I got all these grand things in me, and America won't let me give nothing."

Her teacher, bewildered by such a rush of words, could do nothing but murmur rather lamely: "I think you will have to go elsewhere if you want to set the world on fire." But that is not really what Anzia Yezierska was driving at; it was only in properly sublimated literary form that she wished to set the world on fire. She wanted to write books, stories, novels, an autobiography. She wished to give vent to the impulses to self-expression which had been bottled up inside her until she got here. And eventually, it must be said, she had her way. Like the child who, according to Emerson in his essay *Self-Reliance,* by a steadfast refusal to conform to others turns the adults around him into children and makes them conform to him, she had her say in her own way.

She never became more than almost famous (and to be almost famous is about as consoling as to wind up with the second-best hand in a poker game), and then the result had been achieved less by her own talents than by the relentless grinding of Hollywood publicity mills over a number of years. These mills, unlike those of the gods, do not grind very fine, and they projected a false image of her into the public mind for a while. She never became very wealthy either, though for a time before the Depression of 1929 she could probably have been described with accuracy as well-to-do. But it was something after all for her to speak out freely to the world; even the "higher-ups" in America (as she naïvely called them) were compelled to listen to her attentively for a time. Her observations and messages are incorporated into half a dozen little books and several uncollected articles. These are mostly still readable and continue to be of interest, which is more than can be said of many of the literary productions—not to speak of the more ephemeral journalism— which came into the world at the same time as her own.

Red Ribbon on a White Horse

I paused in front of my rooming house on Hester Street. This was 1920, when Hester Street was the pushcart center of the East Side. The air reeked with the smell of fish and overripe fruit from the carts in front of the house. I peeked into the basement window. The landlady was not there to nag me for the rent. I crept into her kitchen, filled my pitcher with water and hurried out. In my room I set the kettle boiling. There wasn't much taste to the stale tea leaves but the hot water warmed me. I was still sipping my tea, thankful for this short reprieve from my landlady, when I heard my name shouted outside the door.

The angel of death, I thought, my landlady had come to put me out! And Hester Street had gathered to watch another eviction. I opened the door with fear.

Mrs. Katz with her baby in her arms, Mrs. Rubin drying her wet hands on her apron, and Zalmon Shlomoh, the fish peddler, crowded into my room, pushing forward a Western Union messenger who handed me a yellow envelope.

"*Oi-oi weh!* A telegram!" Mrs. Rubin wailed. "Somebody died?"

Their eyes gleamed with prying curiosity. "Read—read already!" they clamored.

I ripped open the envelope and read:

TELEPHONE IMMEDIATELY FOR AN APPOINTMENT TO DISCUSS MOTION PICTURE RIGHTS OF "HUNGRY HEARTS"

R. L. GIFFEN

Selection from Anzia Yezierska's *Red Ribbon on a White Horse*, published by Charles Scribner's Sons, New York, 1950.

"Who died?" they demanded.

"Nobody died. It's only a place for a job," I said, shooing them out of the room.

I reread the message. "Telephone immediately!" It was from one of the big moving-picture agents. In those days Hollywood was still busy with Westerns and Pollyanna romances. The studios seldom bought stories from life. This was like winning a ticket on a lottery.

Hungry Hearts had been my first book. It had been praised by the critics, esteemed as literature. That meant it didn't sell. After spending the two hundred dollars I had received in royalties, I was even poorer than when I had started writing.

And now movie rights! Money! Wealth! I could get the world for the price of a telephone call. But if I had had a nickel for a telephone I wouldn't have fooled a starving stomach with stewed-over tea leaves. I needed a nickel for telephoning, ten cents for carfare—fifteen cents! What could I pawn to get fifteen cents?

I looked about my room. The rickety cot didn't belong to me. The rusty gas plate on the window sill? My typewriter? The trunk that was my table? Then I saw the shawl, my mother's shawl that served as a blanket and a cover for my cot.

Nobody in our village in Poland had had a shawl like it. It had been Mother's wedding present from her rich uncle in Warsaw. It had been her Sabbath, her holiday. . . . When she put it on she outshone all the other women on the way to the synagogue.

Old and worn—it held memories of my childhood, put space and color in my drab little room. It redeemed the squalor in which I had to live. But this might be the last time I'd have to pawn it. I seized the shawl and rushed with it to the pawnshop.

Zaretzky, the pawnbroker, was a bald-headed dwarf, grown gray with the years in the dark basement—tight-skinned and crooked from squeezing pennies out of despairing people.

I watched his dirty, bony fingers appraise the shawl. "An old rag!" he grunted, peering at me through his thick-rimmed glasses. He had always intimidated me before, but this time the telegram in my hand made me bold.

"See here, Zaretzky," I said, "this shawl is rarer than diamonds—an antique from Poland, pure wool. The older it gets, the finer—the softer the colors—"

He spread it out and held it up to the light. "A moth-eaten rag full of holes!"

"You talk as if I were a new customer. You make nothing of the best things. As you did with my samovar."

"A samovar is yet something. But this!" He pushed the shawl from him. "A quarter. Take it or leave it."

"This was the finest shawl in Plinsk. It's hand-woven, hand-dyed. People's lives are woven into it."

"For what is past nobody pays. Now it's junk—falling apart."

"I'm only asking a dollar. It's worth ten times that much. Only a dollar!"

"A quarter. You want it? Yes or no?"

I grabbed the quarter and fled.

Within a half-hour I was at the agent's office.

"I've great news for you," he said, drawing up a chair near his desk. "I've practically sold your book to Hollywood. Goldwyn wants it. Fox is making offers, too, but I think Goldwyn is our best bet. They offered five thousand dollars. I'm holding out for ten."

I had pawned Mother's shawl to get there, and this man talked of thousands of dollars. Five, ten thousand dollars was a fortune in 1920. I was suddenly aware of my hunger. I saw myself biting into thick, juicy steaks, dipping fresh rolls into mounds of butter, swallowing whole platters of French fried potatoes in one gulp.

"If we settle with Goldwyn," Mr. Giffen said, "He will want you to go to Hollywood to collaborate on the script."

I stood up to go, dizzy from lack of food and so much excitement.

"'Maybe what you're saying is real," I said. "If it is, then can you advance me one dollar on all these thousands?"

Smiling, he handed me a bill.

I walked out of his office staring at the ten-dollar bill in my hand. Directly across the street was the white-tiled front of a Childs restaurant. How often I had stood outside this same restaurant, watching the waitresses clear away leftover food and wanting to cry out, "Don't throw it away! Give it to me. I'm hungry!" I stumbled through the door, sank into the first vacant chair and ordered the most expensive steak on the menu. A

270

platter was set before me—porterhouse steak, onions, potatoes, rolls, butter. I couldn't eat fast enough. Before I was half through, my throat tightened. My head bent over my plate, tears rolled down my cheeks onto the uneaten food.

When I hadn't had a penny for a roll I had had the appetite of a wolf that could devour the earth. Now that I could treat myself to a dollar dinner, I couldn't take another bite. But just having something to eat, even though I could only half eat it, made me see the world with new eyes. If only Father and Mother were alive now! How I longed to be at peace with them!

I had not meant to abandon them when I left home—I had only wanted to get to the place where I belonged. To do it, I had to strike out alone.

If my mother could only have lived long enough to see that I was not the heartless creature I seemed to be! As for my father— would he forgive me even now?

Now that there was no longer reason to feel sorry for myself, my self-pity turned to regret for all that I did not do and might have done for them.

The waitress started to remove the dishes.

"I'm not through!" I held onto the plate, still starved for the steak and potatoes I could not eat. The agent's talk of Hollywood might have been only a dream. But steak was real. When no one was looking, I took out my handkerchief, thrust the meat and cold potatoes into it, covered it with my newspaper and sneaked out like a thief with the food for which I had paid.

Back in my room I opened the newspaper bundle, still too excited with the prospect of Hollywood to be able to eat. "God! What a hoarding creature I've become!" I cried out in self-disgust. In my purse was the change from the ten-dollar bill the agent had given me. More than enough for a dozen meals. And yet the hoarding habit of poverty was so deep in my bones that I had to bring home the food that I could not eat.

I leaned out of the window. Lily, the alley cat, was scavenging the garbage can as usual. I had named her Lily because she had nothing but garbage to eat and yet somehow looked white and beautiful like the lilies that rise out of dunghills.

"Lily!" I called to her, holding up the steak. The next moment she bounded up on my window sill, devouring the steak and potatoes in huge gulps.

"I've been a pauper all my life," I told Lily as I watched her eat. "But I'll be a pauper no longer. I'll have money, plenty of it. I'll not only have money to buy food when I'm hungry, but I'll have men who'll love me on my terms. An end to hoarding food, or hoarding love!"

I threw open the trunk, dug down and yanked out the box of John Morrow's letters, determined to tear them up and shed the memory of them once and for all. For years those letters had been to me music and poetry. I had stayed up nights to console my loneliness reading and rereading them, drugged with the opiate of his words.

But now, with the prospect of Hollywood, I began to hate those letters. Why hang on to words when the love that had inspired them was dead? In Hollywood there would be new people. There would be other men.

I seized the first letter and began tearing it. But a panicky fear of loss stopped me. Money could buy meat and mink, rye bread and rubies, but not the beauty of his words. Those letters were my assurance that I was a woman who could love and be loved. Without them, I was again the oddity of Hester Street, an object of pity and laughter.

"Poor thing! I can't stand the starved-dog look in her eyes," I had overheard one of the men in the shop say to another.

"Well, if you're so sorry for her, marry her," came the jeering retort.

"Marry her? Oi-i-i! Oi-yoi! That *meshugeneh?* That redheaded witch? Her head is on wheels, riding on air. She's not a woman. She has a *dybbuk,* a devil, a book for a heart."

But when I met John Morrow, the *dybbuk* that drove away other men had drawn him to me. He saw my people in me, struggling for a voice. I could no more tear up those letters than I could root out the memory of him!

I slipped the torn pieces of the letter into the envelope, put it back with the others in the box and stuck it at the bottom of my trunk, under my old clothes.

A week later Mr. Giffen asked me to lunch to talk over the movie contract I was to sign.

After I had signed a twenty-page contract, Giffen handed me a check—a check made out to me—a check for nine thousand dollars.

"I've deducted one thousand for my ten per cent," he explained.

I looked at the check. Nine thousand dollars!

"Riches for a lifetime!" I cried.

Giffen smiled. "It's only the beginning. When you're in Hollywood you'll see the more you have, the more you'll get."

He took out my railroad reservation from his wallet and handed it to me. "They want you to assist in the production of the book. You're to get two hundred a week and all your expenses while there."

He gave me another check for a hundred dollars. "This is for your incidentals on the train. Meals for three and a half days—one hundred dollars. Not so bad!" He patted my hand. "Young lady! You go on salary the moment you step on the train."

I told him I could be ready as soon as I got something out of a pawnshop.

With my purse full of money, I hurried to Zaretzky's to redeem my shawl.

"Zaretzky!" I charged into the basement. "I forgot to take my receipt for the shawl!"

"Forgot nothing! I gave it to you in your hand."

"I swear to you, I left it on the counter."

"If you were crazy enough to lose it, it's not my fault."

I took out a five-dollar bill. "Here's five dollars for your quarter," I said. "What more do you want?"

He made no move. He stood like stone staring at me.

"Shylock! Here's ten dollars! I have no time to bargain with you. If that's not enough, here's twice ten dollars! Twenty dollars for your twenty-five cents!"

There was a flicker in the black pinpoints of his eyes. He took out a signed receipt from the money box. "I sold it the day you brought it here for five dollars," he groaned, his face distorted by frustrated greed.

The next day I packed my belongings without the shawl that had gone with me everywhere I went. The loss of that one beautiful thing which all my money could not reclaim shadowed my prospective trip to Hollywood.

The distrust of good fortune always in the marrow of my bones made me think of my father. While I was struggling with hunger and want, trying to write, I feared to go near him. I couldn't stand his condemnation of my lawless, godless, selfish existence. But now, with Hollywood ahead of me, I had the courage to face him. As I entered the dark hallway of the tenement where he lived, I heard his voice chanting.

"And a man shall be as a hiding place from the wind, and covert from the tempest; as rivers of water in a dry place, as the shadow of a great rock in a weary land. . . ."

Since earliest childhood I had heard this chant of Isaiah. It was as familiar to me as Mother Goose rhymes to other children. Hearing it again after so many years, I was struck for the first time by the beauty of the words. Though my father was poor and had nothing, the Torah, the poetry of prophets, was his daily bread.

He was still chanting as I entered, a gray-bearded man in a black skullcap.

"And the eyes of them that see shall not be dim, and the ears of them that hear shall hearken. The heart of the rash shall understand knowledge, and the tongue of the stammerers shall be ready to speak plainly. . . ."

As I stood there, waiting for him to see me, I noticed the aging stoop of his shoulders. He was getting paler, thinner. The frail body accused me for having been away so long. But in the same moment of guilt the smells of the musty room in which he wouldn't permit a window to be opened or a book to be dusted made me want to run. On the table piled high with his papers and dust-laden books were dishes with remains of his last meal—cabbage soup and pumpernickel. He was as unaware of the squalor around him as a medieval monk.

Dimly I realized that this new world didn't want his kind. He had no choice but to live for God. And I, his daughter, who abandoned him for the things of this world, had joined the world against him.

He looked up and saw me.

"So you've come at last? You've come to see your old father?"

"I was so busy . . ." I mumbled. And then, hastily, to halt his reproaches, I reached into my bag and dropped ten ten-dollar bills on the open page of his book. He pushed aside the bills as if they would contaminate the holiness of the script.

"Months, almost a year, you've been away. . . ."

"Bessie, Fannie live right near here, they promised to look after you. . . ."

"They have their own husbands to look after. You're my only unmarried daughter. Your first duty to God is to serve your father. But what's an old father to an *Amerikanerin*, a daughter of Babylon?"

"Your daughter of Babylon brought you a hundred dollars."

"Can your money make up for your duty as a daughter? In America, money takes the place of God."

"But I earned that money with my writing." For all his scorn of my godlessness, I thought he would take a father's pride in my success. "Ten thousand they paid me. . . ."

He wouldn't let me finish. He shook a warning finger in my face. "Can you touch pitch without being defiled? Neither can you hold on to all that money without losing your soul."

Even in the street, his words still rang in my ears. "Daughter of Babylon! You've polluted your inheritance. . . . You'll wander in darkness and none shall be there to save you. . . ."

His old God could not save me in a new world, I told myself. Why did we come to America, if not to achieve all that had been denied us for centuries in Europe? Fear and poverty were behind me. I was going into a new world of plenty. I would learn to live in the now . . . not in the next world.

I had but to open my purse, look at my reservation for a drawing room on the fastest flyer to Hollywood, think of the fabulous salary I was to be paid even while traveling, and no hope in which I might indulge was too high, no longing too visionary.

Grand Central Station, where I waited for my train, seemed an unreal place. Within the vast marble structure people rushed in and out, meeting, parting and hurrying on, each in pursuit of his own dream. As I stood lost in my thoughts, every man I saw seemed John Morrow coming to see me off. If so incredible a thing could happen as my going to Hollywood, surely John Morrow could appear. He must know *Hungry Hearts* was written for him. He must sense my need to share my wealth with him even more than I had needed him in poverty.

The gates opened. My train was called. I picked up my bundle, started through the gate, still looking back, still expecting the miracle. I could not give up the hope that love as great as his had been could ever cease.

The first days and nights on the train I was too dazed by the sudden turn of events to notice the view from my window. Miles of beautiful country I saw, unaware of what I was seeing. Then one morning I woke up and saw the desert stretching out on both sides. The train raced through the wide monotonous landscape at a terrific pace to reach its destination on scheduled time.

It was getting hotter and hotter. Sand sifted through the screened air vents and closed doors. The train stopped at the station to refuel. Passengers stepped out to buy trinkets from the Indians squatting on the platform. Over the entrance of an adobe building I read in gilt letters the inscription:

THE DESERT WAITED, SILENT AND HOT AND FIERCE IN ITS DESOLATION, HOLDING ITS TREASURES UNDER SEAL OF DEATH AGAINST THE COMING OF THE STRONG ONE.

I looked across the vast space and thought of the time when all this silent sand was a rolling ocean. What eons had to pass for the ocean to dry into this arid waste! In the immensity of the desert the whirl of trivialities which I had so magnified all fell away. I was suspended in timelessness—sand, sky, and space. What a relief it was to let go—not to think—not to feel, but rest, silent—past, present and future stretching to infinity.

Slowly, imperceptibly, the dry desert air receded before the humid, subtropical warmth of southern California. The sense of time and the concern with self stirred again. Green hills, dazzling gardens and orange groves, towering date palms ushered in the great adventure ahead of me.

At the Los Angeles station I was met by a man who introduced himself as Mr. Irving Lenz, chief of Goldwyn's publicity department.

"Where's your baggage?" he asked.

I pointed to my bundles. There had been no time to buy luggage or anything else.

In the midst of the crowd coming and going to the trains I found myself surrounded by curious-eyed men and women. Pencils and notebooks were pulled out, cameras opened.

"Who are all these people?" I asked.

"Reporters to interview you," Lenz said.

They stared at me as if I were some strange animal on the way to the zoo.

"To what do you attribute your success?" one of the reporters began.

I looked at him. For days and nights I had been whirled in a Niagara of unreality, wondering what it was all about. And he asked for a formula of success.

"What are you going to do with all your money?" another went on.

While I stood panic-stricken, tongue-tied, cameras clicked, flashlights exploded.

"Take me out of this," I appealed to Mr. Lenz.

"Why, this is part of the game," Lenz laughed. "A million-dollar build-up for your book."

With the cameras still clicking, he took my arm and led me to an automobile.

In one of those limousines which I had always condemned as a criminal luxury, I was driven to the Miramar Hotel. A basket of roses greeted me when I walked into my apartment. No one had ever put flowers in a room for me before. I lifted the roses high in the air, then hugged them to me.

There was a knock at the door. A maid in black and white came in. "Does Madame wish any help in unpacking? Or perhaps in dressing for dinner?"

I was wearing the only clothes I had—blue serge skirt and cotton blouse bought at a basement bargain counter. They were rumpled from travel.

"No, no, I need nothing," I stammered.

With one swift glance she appraised the cheapness and rough-
ness of my clothes and withdrew.

As the door closed behind her, I walked into the bedroom.
More flowers. I touched the bed. Clean, soft, smooth. I lifted the
bedspread, feasting my eyes on the white sheets, the wool blankets. Who could lie down and disturb this delicate perfection?

Another door. Bathtub, washbowl, and toilet. My own. White-
tiled walls. Sunlight streaming in through clean, glass windows.
Racks with towels—towels big as blankets, bath towels, hand
towels. Bath salts in crystal bottles. Soap wrapped in silver foil.
Toilet paper, canary-colored to match the towels.

I looked down for the imprint of my shoes on the white-tiled
floor. How could I desecrate the cleanliness of that tub with my
dirty body? I thought of the hours I had to stand in line at the
public bathhouse before Passover and the New Year—and the
greasy tub smelling of the sweat of the crowd. The iron sink in
the hall on Hester Street. One faucet for eight families. Here were
two faucets. Hot water, cold water, all the water in the world. I
turned on both faucets and let them run for the sheer joy of it.

I danced across the fawn-colored carpet in the sitting room
and flopped down into one easy chair after another. Then up and
out to the balcony, down the terrace to the private beach washed
by the ocean waves. I looked at the shimmering water dotted with
white yachts. The Atlantic led back to Poland. The Pacific
stretched to the home of Kubla Khan.

It was too big, too beautiful. Could I ever get used to living in
such comfort? Could I enjoy such affluence unless I could forget
the poverty back of me? Forget? The real world, the tenement
where I had lived, blotted out the sun and sky. I saw myself, a
scrawny child of twelve, always hungry, always asking questions.
It was soon after we had come to America. We lived on Hester
Street in a railroad flat that was always dark. One morning my
mother was in the kitchen, bent over the washtub, rubbing
clothes.

"When was I born?" I asked, pulling her apron. "When is my
birthday?"

She gave no sign that she had heard me.

"Minnie, the janitor's daughter, will have a party. A cake with candles on it for a birthday. All children have birthdays. Everybody on the block knows her age but me." I pounded the table with my fist. "I must have a birthday like other children."

"Birthdays?" Mother stopped washing and looked at me, her eyes black with gloom. "A birthday wills itself in you? What is with you the great joy? No shirt on your back—no shoes on your feet—not a penny in the house to buy bread—and you want yet birthdays? The landlord's daughter can have birthdays. For her, the music plays. For her, life is a feast. For you—a funeral. Bury yourself in ashes and weep because you were born in this world."

Like a driven horse feeling the whip behind him, she rubbed the clothes savagely.

"Have you a father like other fathers? Does his wife or his children lay in his head?" Mother wiped the sweat from her face with a heavy hand. "Woe is me! Your father worked for God and His Torah like other fathers work for their wives and children. You ought to light a black candle on your birthday. You ought to lie on your face and cry and curse the day you were born!"

The black curse of poverty followed me during my brief, few days in an American school. I had walked into the classroom without knowing a word of English. The teacher was talking to the children. They knew what she was saying and I knew nothing. I felt like the village idiot in my immigrant clothes so different from the clothes of the other children. But more than the difference of appearance was the unfamiliar language. The sound of every foreign word hammered into me: You'll never know, you'll never learn. . . . And before I could learn, poverty thrust me into the sweatshop.

But that was long ago. Now the sun was shining, laughing at my fears. For the first time in my life I had every reason to be happy. I had pushed my way up out of the darkness into light. I had earned my place in the sun. No backward glances! I would shed the very thought of poverty as I had shed my immigrant's shawl. I had learned to abase myself; now I would learn to lift up my head and look the world in the face.

To begin with, I would eat in state in the dining room. I had no clothes for the occasion. But I was too happy to care about my appearance. My shirtwaist and skirt would have to do.

The headwaiter led me to a central table. Music, soft lights, the gleam of silver and glass on snowy linen. Never had I seen such a shimmer of lovely gowns.

I picked up the gilded menu. What a feast! Ten entrées, a dozen roasts, twice as many desserts. Breaking my resolve to forget, I thought of the blocks I used to walk for stale bread to save two cents. The way I bargained at the pushcarts when the Friday rush was over to get the leftover herring a penny cheaper.

And now—choose! Gorge yourself on Terrine de Pâté de Foie Gras, Green Turtle Soup au Sherry, Jumbo Pigeon on Toast, Canapé Royale Princesse—whatever that is! Choose!

The waiter smiled at me as if he had read my thoughts, and offered me the evening papers. "Your office sent them."

I glanced at the headlines: "Immigrant Wins Fortune in Movies." "Sweatshop Cinderella at the Miramar Hotel." "From Hester Street to Hollywood."

There was a picture of me above those captions, but I couldn't recognize myself in it, any more than I could recognize my own life in the newspapers' stories of my "success."

$$* * * * * * *$$

The following passage is from the concluding chapter of Miss Yezierska's book, which deals with her belated and futile attempt, after a variety of adventures had brought her back from riches to povery, to settle down in a small New England town.

The train from Fair Oaks carried me to an uncertain future, but Mrs. Cobb's farewell at the station had left me on the crest of courage. While I was living there, I hadn't realized how profoundly she had given me of herself, her imagination, her understanding. From the first she had accepted me for what I was, not for anything I had ever done. And so she rekindled in me the vital sense of myself that I had lost when I fled Hester Street. She was as close to me there in the coach as if I were having Sunday breakfast with her in her kitchen. In my lap was the lunch she had prepared—sandwiches, cake, and fruit in neat parcels of waxed paper—a reminder of the warmth and generosity of a prim New England farm woman, the poet of the town, whose greatest poem was herself.

There had always been something haunting in Mrs. Cobb's face. Something that made me feel I had known her somewhere, known her for a long time. And now, on the train, it came to me where I had seen that look before. That expression at once serene and wise had been on my father's face.

The likeness shocked me. The idea that there could be any-thing in common between this reticent New England farm woman and the uncompromising, Old World Jew seemed preposterous. And yet—I scanned their features in memory trying to see what made them alike. The same purity and trustfulness was in their faces. The same "devotion to something afar from the sphere of our sorrow" looked out of their eyes.

A memory I had been pushing aside for years came back to me. It was just after *Bread Givers* was published. I felt I had justified myself in the book for having hardened my heart to go through life alone. I described how my sisters, who had married according to my father's will, spent themselves childbearing in poverty. I too had children. My children were the people I wrote about. I gave my children, born of loneliness, as much of my life as my married sisters did in bringing their children into the world.

The pride in the new book filled me with a longing to see my father. Because I had fought him and broken away from him as a child, I was drawn to him as an adult, now that I was achieving my own place in the world. I felt good, magnanimous. Instead of sending him the usual monthly check by mail, I wanted to give it to him as a token of peace and so forget the terrible fights that had driven me from home.

I found him in his room, bent over the table with his books, his prayer shawl and phylacteries. He closed the Bible and peered at me.

"What is it I hear? You wrote a book about me?" His voice and the sorrow in his eyes left me speechless. "How could you write about someone you don't know?"

"I know you," I mumbled.

"Woe to America!" he wailed. "Only in America could it happen—an ignorant thing like you—a writer! What do you know of life? Of history, philosophy? What do you know of the Bible, the foundation of all knowledge?"

He stood up, an ancient patriarch condemning unrighteousness. His black skullcap set off his white hair and beard. "If you only knew how deep is your ignorance—"

"What have you ever done with all your knowledge?" I demanded. "While you prayed and gloried in your Torah, your children were in the factory, slaving for bread."

His God-kindled face towered over me. "What? Should I have sold my religion? God is not for sale. God comes before my own flesh and blood."

The eyes under the deeply furrowed brow retained the purity of a child and the zeal of a man in love with God all the days of his life. As I looked at him, I was struck by the radiance that the evils of the world could not mar. I envied his inward peace as a homeless one envies the sight of home.

"My child!" His eyes sought mine, as if something in me had touched him. "It says in the Torah: He who separates himself from people buries himself in death. A woman alone, not a wife and not a mother, has no existence. No joy on earth, no hope of heaven.

"Look around you. Nothing in nature lives alone. The birds in the air, the fishes in the sea, even the worms under the stone need their own kind to fulfill themselves."

The uselessness of my visit! Each time I came to see him, he reminded me that I was unmarried and attacked me for my godlessness. His Old World preaching drained the joy out of my life. The more we tried to reach each other, the deeper grew the gulf between us.

"You're not human!" he went on. "Can the Ethiopian change his skin, or the leopard his spots? Neither can good come from your evil worship of Mammon. Woe! Woe! Your barren heart looks out from your eyes."

His words were salt on my wounds. In desperation, I picked up purse and gloves and turned toward the door.

"I see you're in a hurry, all ready to run away. Run! Where?

282

For what? To get a higher place in the Tower of Babel? To make more money out of your ignorance?

"Poverty becomes a Jew like a red ribbon on a white horse. But you're no longer a Jew. You're a *meshumeides,* an apostate, an enemy of your own people. And even the Christians will hate you."

I fled from him in anger and resentment. But it was no use. I could never escape him. He was the conscience that condemned me. "Can fire and water be together? Neither can truth be in the market place. Truth grows in silence, in stillness, in the secret place of the Most High—not in sounding brass and tinkling cymbals. . . ."

Now, all these years after his death, the ideas he tried to force on me revealed their meaning. Again and again at crucial turning points of my life, his words flared out of the darkness. "He who separates himself from people buries himself in death. . . . Can fire and water be together? Neither can godliness and the flesh-pots of Mammon. . . . Poverty becomes a Jew. . . ." He didn't feel himself poor. Poverty had never starved him as it had me. Having nothing only drew him closer to God. Homelessness, hunger, exile—Jews had survived them for thousands of years. What was there to fear in a shabby coat? He walked the earth knowing that the "kingdom, the power, and the glory" were in his own heart; and no worldly prizes could swerve him from his chosen path.

But this single-mindedness, this immunity to the changes around him—this strength was also his limitation. He ignored the world I had to live in and compromise with. Centuries yawned between us.

It was Mrs. Cobb who brought me back to him. She was like a still pool in whose depth I caught a glimpse of the self from which I had been fleeing. With new-opened eyes I saw the poverty of spirit that had kept me barren till now, the fierce obsession of my will to lift my head up out of the squalor and anonymity of the poor.

Years ago, in Hollywood, Samuel Goldwyn said to me that to tell a good story, you must know the end before you begin it. And if you know the end, you can sum up the whole plot in a sentence. But I had always plunged into writing before I knew where it would take me. If a story was alive, it worked itself out as I wrote it. Even when I began this story, long before I went to Fair Oaks, I did not know how it would end—that is, the meaning of the end. I thought I was writing the downward career of a failure. Goldwyn would have summed it up in a phrase: "From an author in Hollywood to a pauper on W.P.A."

I wanted to unburden my shame for having failed. But on the train as I faced my disgrace, I saw that Hollywood was not my success, nor my present poverty and anonymity, failure. I saw that "success," "failure," "poverty," "riches," were price tags, money values of the market place which had mesmerized and sidetracked me for years.

For a long time I sat still, staring at the passing scenery through which the train was speeding, pondering the loneliness in each individual soul. The struggle of man, alone with the feeble resources of courage at his command, against a universe that cares nothing for his hopes and fears.

I remembered a dream I had had the night before. I was on a train just like this one. People were getting off at various stations, but I didn't know where to get off, my mind became a blank. As the conductor approached for the fare, I saw I had lost my purse and I cried out, "Oh, my God! I have no money and I don't know where I'm going!"

The anxiety that had hounded me from the day I was born was ready to pounce on me again. It had kept me on the run all my life. Even when I came to Fair Oaks I was running, but I couldn't escape it. The ghetto was with me wherever I went—the nothingness, the fear of my nothingness. Marian Foster had given me all that could be given a beggar—a house, chattels, milk, bread— while I resented her for withholding what she could not give, the understanding that I thought would make me secure. I had sought security in the mud and in the stars, sought it in the quick riches and glory of Hollywood and in the security wage of W.P.A. I sought it everywhere but in myself. Suddenly I felt like that ship-wrecked sailor who had been picked up, dying of thirst, unaware that the current into which he had drifted was fresh water.

A warm wave of happiness welled up in me. Often before I

had tried to be happy, but this happiness now came unbidden, unwilled, as though all the hells I had been through had opened a secret door. Why had I no premonition in the wandering years when I was hungering and thirsting for recognition, that this quiet joy, this sanctuary, was waiting for me after I had sunk back to anonymity? I did not have to go to far places, sweat for glory, strain for the smile from important people. All that I could ever be, the glimpses of truth I reached for everywhere, was in myself.

The power that makes grass grow, fruit ripen, and guides the bird in its flight is in us all. At any moment when man becomes aware of that inner power, he can rise above the accidents of fortune that rule his outward life, creating and recreating himself out of his defeats.

Yesterday I was a bungler, an idiot, a blind destroyer of myself, reaching for I knew not what and only pushing it from me in my ignorance. Today the knowledge of a thousand failures cannot keep me from this light born of my darkness, here, now.

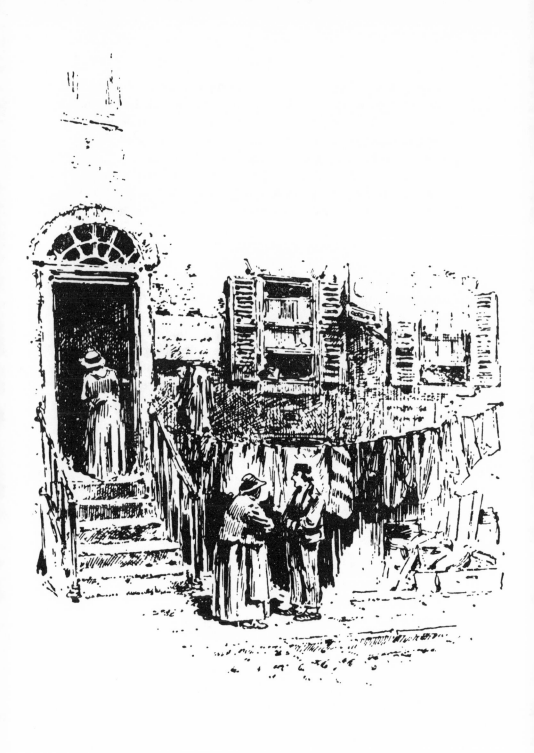

JAMES GIBBONS HUNEKER

James Gibbons Huneker, who is described in the reference work *Twentieth Century Authors* as an art and music critic as well as a "miscellaneous writer," was born in Philadelphia on Januray 31, 1860, the son of John H. Huneker, a well-to-do businessman who was an amateur botanist, who collected etchings, and presided over a salon in his home in which many celebrities were entertained. His mother, Mary, was the daughter of the Irish poet James Gibbons. The Huneker family was of Hungarian origin but had been in America since 1700.

James was sent as a child to Roth's Military Academy in Philadelphia but disliked discipline imposed from without as much as Poe did and had to be taken out by his parents at the age of twelve. More to his taste were theaters and museums which he frequented with a passionate attachment. By temperament, he was apparently something of an autodidact and undertook of his own volition a vast program of reading. Only in music did he submit enthusiastically to formal training and he studied in Philadelphia with two piano teachers, one of whom had been a pupil of Chopin and the other of Liszt. He also played the organ well enough to be hired by a Jewish temple to play on Saturdays, while on Sundays his services went to a Catholic church.

In 1881, at the age of twenty-one, he came to New York City in the role of critic and journalist. He also continued his music lessons there with the famous pianist Joseffy. For the next fifteen years he wrote for the *Musical Courier*. He pursued his various activities energetically; in his own words, he lived luxuriously and worked like a dog. In 1900, he published a book called *Chopin:*

The Man and His Work, which established his reputation. He also edited Chopin's piano music. He travelled much in Europe, visiting the theaters, art shrines, and concert halls in connection with his professional interests but also because he was, as he called himself, "a travel maniac." Of all the cities in Europe which he visited, Bruges appears to have been his favorite.

Of his critical influence in America, exercised through the many journalistic articles which he regularly wrote and which were just as regularly collected into books after his reputation as a writer was made, H. L. Mencken said: "It would be difficult, indeed, to overestimate the practical value to all the arts in America of his intellectual alertness, his catholic hospitality to ideas, his artistic courage, and above all, his powers of persuasion." Like some other well-known critics in literary history, he seems to have shone more brilliantly in conversation than he did in writing, about which *Twentieth Century Authors* justly remarks: "His literary method is somewhat spasmodic and disjointed; sentence following sentence, not always in logical sequence." His portrait of the East Side is one of the most eccentrically individualistic ones that I have found anywhere and fairly represents, I think, both his talent and its limitations, which over the years must have caused him to puzzle at least as many readers as he has pleased.

He died on February 9, 1921. Since then, the affection of notable friends like Mencken has been instrumental in bringing some of his books back into print, and he has also been made the subject of some academic studies. He has found a place, however modest, in the cultural history of the United States.

The New Cosmopolis: A Book of Images

The illusions of the middle-aged die hardest. At twenty I discovered, with sorrow, that there was no such enchanted spot as the Latin Quarter. An old Frenchman with whom I dined daily at that time in a luxurious Batignolles gargote informed me that Paris had seen the last of the famous quarter after the Commune, but a still older person who wrote obituary notices for the parish swore the Latin Quarter had not been in existence since 1848; the swelling tide of democracy had swept away the darling superstitions of the students, many of whom became comfortably rich when Napoleon the Little grasped the crown. This I set down as pure legend. Had I not seen young painters, poets, and musicians in baggy velvet trousers walk up and down the Boul' Mich' during the Exposition of 1878? And they still pranced about the cafés and brasseries in 1914, their hair as long as their thirst. There may be no Latin Quarter, but the Latin Quarter is ever in a young man's soul who goes to Paris in pursuit of the golden fleece of art.

I recovered from the disillusionment and no more bothered my head about this pasteboard Bohemia than I did at the island of Marken when I was told that its Dutch peasants with their picturesque costumes and head-dress were moonshine manufactured by an enterprising travel bureau to attract tourists. Are there not more Puritans in the West than in New England? But the loss of such a treasured illusion as our own East Side smote me severely. When young and buoyant, one illusion crowds out another, After you have crossed the great divide of fifty, with the mountains of

Selection from *The New Cosmopolis: A Book of Images* by James Huneker, published by Scribner's, New York, 1915.

the moon behind you, and an increasing waist measurement before you, the annulment of a cherished image wounds the soul.

The East Side with its Arabian Nights entertainment was such an image. Twenty years ago you could play the rôle of the disguised Sultan and with a favourite Vizier sally forth at eve from Park Row in pursuit of strange adventures. What thrilling encounters! What hairbreadth escapes! What hand-to-hand struggles with genii, afrits, imps—bottle-imps, very often—dangerous bandits, perilous policemen and nymphs or thrice dangerous anarchists! To slink down an ill-lighted, sinister alley full of Chinese and American tramps, to hurry by solitary policemen as if engaged in some criminal enterprise, to enter the abode of them that never wash, where bad beer and terrible tobacco filled the air with discordant perfumes—ah! what joys for adventurous souls, what tremendous dawns over Williamsburg, what glorious headaches were ours on awakening the next night! An East Side there was in those hardy times, and it was still virginal to settlement-workers, sociological cranks, impertinent reformers, self-advertising politicians, billionaire socialists, and the ubiquitous newspaper man. Magazine writers had not topsyturvied the ideas of the tenement dwellers, nor were the street-cleaner, the Board of Health, and other destroyers of the picturesque in evidence. It was the dear old dirty, often disreputable, though never dull East Side; while now the sentimentalist feels a heart pang to see the order, the cleanliness, the wide streets, the playgrounds, the big boulevards, the absence of indigence that have spoiled the most interesting part of New York City.

Well I remember the night, years ago, when finding ourselves in Tompkins Square we went across to Justus Schwab's and joined an anarchist meeting in full swing. There were no bombs, though there was plenty of beer. A more amiable and better-informed man than Schwab never trod carpet slippers. The discussions in German and English betrayed a culture not easily duplicated on the West Side—wherever that mysterious territory really is. Before Nietzsche's and Stirner's names were pronounced in our lecture-rooms they were familiarly quoted at Schwab's. By request I played The Marseillaise and The International Hymn on an old piano—smoke-stained, with rattling keys and a cracked tone—which stood at the rear upon a platform. All was peace and a flow of soul; yet the place was raided before midnight and a band of indignant, also merry, prisoners marched to the police station. Naturally no one was detained but Schwab. The police felt called upon to arrest somebody around Tompkins Square about once a month. ANARCHIST OUTRAGES was the usual newspaper headline. Why are the Mafia performers never called anarchs? To-day the Black Hand terrorises a region where the bombs in the old times were manufactured of ink for the daily papers. They generally blow themselves up, these anarchists; but there is nothing adventurous in having an eye or a leg blown away by a Sicilian you have never seen. To be arrested twenty years ago for the romantic crime of playing The Marseillaise on a badly tuned piano—is it any wonder I get sentimental when I think of an East Side that is no more? Perhaps the younger generation, which Ibsen described as "knocking," may have its nooks unknown to us, but the old fascination has flown.

Yet like the war-horse that is put out to grass and rears when it hears the tin dinner horn, we pricked ears on learning one summer afternoon that up on First Avenue there was a wonderful brew of beer to be had. Pilsner beer served across genuine Bohemian tables! How the rumour came to my ears I've forgotten, but I was not long in sending its glad import over the telephone. Remember that we now dwell in a city where never before has so much badly kept beer been sold. The show-places are gaudy and Americanised. Fashionable slummers whose fathers wore leathern aprons and drank their beer from tin pails sip champagne at some noisy gilded cabarets or summer gardens to the banging and scraping of fake gipsy orchestras. Where are the small old-fashioned beer saloons of yesteryear with the sanded floor, the pinochle players, and the ripe, pure beverage? Indeed, the German element on the East Side is in the minority. At least it seems so, for your eardrums are pelted by Bohemian, Yiddish, Hun, Italian, Russian, and other tongues. Many speak German, some sort of German, but the original Germans, the Urdeutsch who came to America more than half a century ago, are dead or decaying; their sons and daughters and grandchildren have

moved into more fashionable districts and shudder if you mention the name of Goethe.

At first the Professor demurred. He is not timid, but a creature
of habit. To tell him the news fraught with significance that you
could imbibe foamy nectar while sitting on a high stool in front
of a bar, a real, pleasant Bohemian facing you, your elbows
occasionally joggled by visiting "growlers," did not appeal to my
bookish friend as I had expected. I routed the Painter den, and
by combined assault we carried the Professor uptown.

"Get off," I said, "at Seventy-second Street and walk across to
First Avenue."

We did so. The prosperity of the neighbourhood after we
crossed Third Avenue was positively dispiriting. First Avenue we
discovered to be wider than Broadway. Oddly enough, human
beings like ourselves passed to and fro. It was the hottest hour of
the afternoon. The world in shirt-sleeves sat perched upon steps
or chairs, lounged in doorways watching the multitudinous babies
that rolled over the sidewalk. The east side of the avenue was
deserted, for the sun beat upon the walls and reverberated blind-
ing rays. Of drunkenness we saw none. We were in the Bohemian
quarter. At Sokol Hall on Seventy-third Street there were a few
pool games in progress; no one stood at the bar. I was the
spokesman:

"Isn't there," I said in my choicest Marienbad Bohemian,
"isn't there a remarkable Pilsner Urquell somewhere in this
neighbourhood?"

"We also sell Pilsner," was the Slavic, evasive answer of a
bartender with the mask of a tragic actor.

"Oh, he means Joe's," interrupted a sympathetic bystander.
"Of course, Joe keeps the dandy beer."

To this there would be but one reply. We stood treat to the
house and went to Kasper's, followed at a discreet distance by
several patriots.

By this time the Professor's collar and temper were running a
race for the wilting sweepstakes. Joe was pleased to see us. We
sat on the celebrated high stools at the bar, and Gambrinus would
have been satisfied. It was the essence of Pilsen, Prague, Marienbad, all in a large glass. Joe discoursed. He was proud that we

liked his interpretation of the wet blond masterpiece; but not too proud. You can't spoil Joe. He is a wary and travelled man. His son, born here, he tells you with ill-concealed affection, is a violinist, a pupil at Vienna of Sevic, the great teacher of Kubelik, of Kocian! Who knows whether another K may not be added to this group. We drink his health and venture the hope that the triumph of the youthful Kasper will not put into the head of the father any futile notion of retiring. Art is all very well. Violin virtuosi abound; but few men there are who know the subtle science of keeping beer at a proper temperature.

"Look here," cried the Professor, "this is nice, but how about the East Side that you are going to show us, the East Side which is not in existence?"

I suggested that we were on the East Side, uptown, to be sure, nevertheless East Side.

"I want to see the East Side of George Luks, and please spare us your antiquated memories. George Moore knows how to relate memories of his dead life, but you don't. Let's be going." It was the Professor in his most didactic mood.

The Painter, who was comfortably anchored, sighed profoundly. He didn't need to leave a snug harbour to see the East Side of George Luks. To my remonstrances and heated assertion that there was no more East Side, that it was only a fable, the Professor bristled up like the Celt he is. "What, then, is the use of writing about a thing that no longer exists? Or, as Israel Zangwill asks in the form of a magnificent pun, 'What's the use of being a countess if you have nothing to count?'" This was too much, and in less than an hour we were threading the intricacies of Grand Street, heading for the region of socialistic rainbows.

"They're off!" chuckled the Painter as he drew forth his sketching pad and pencil.

After a tolerably long tramp we turned south. The street was narrow and not too odorous. High buildings on either side were pierced by numerous windows from which hung frowzy ladies, usually with babies at their bosoms; the fire-escapes were crowded with bedclothes, the middle of the street filled with quarrelling children. The national game on a miniature scale was in progress, and on the sidewalks when the pushcart men per-

293

mitted, encouraging voices called aloud in Yiddish to the baseball heroes. I don't know what they said, but I caught such phrases as these: "Yakie! Schlemil! machen Sie dot first base! Esel! Oh, du!" And the little Jacob toiled up the street and down again, sprawling over garbage-cans, upsetting two girls dressed in resplendent ribbons for Shabbas, finally touching an old basket and getting full in his smudged features a soft tomato. "Aus!" yelled the umpire who was immediately kicked in the stomach. "Aus! Out!" came in delirious tones from a dancing mass of men— Jewish men with the traditional whiskers, brown straw hats, and alpaca coats. It was startling even to the Professor.

"There is your twentieth-century East Side for you," I began, but the Painter watched other things.

"Yet they think Luks is too realistic, don't they? Just look at those girls." He pointed out a red-headed Irish girl clutching a blonde girl, unmistakably a German blonde, who were both dreamily waltzing to the faded tune of The Merry Widow.

Music which we hurry from across town is near the East River music the conqueror. It mellows the long hours of dry, dusty summer days, and it sets moving in earnest if not graceful rhythms the legs of the little ones. Suddenly the organ began a gallop. Off whisked the girls—Delia and Marike were their names, we were later informed—off they went like two abandoned spielers disguised as children of poverty. What movement! What fire! The blonde with her silvery locks stamped and whirled off her feet the trim Irish girl with the dark red curls.

"Are you chaps never coming along?" asked the Professor. "It will be night soon, and we haven't seen anything yet."

"He's afraid Mouquin's will close before he gets back to civilization," sardonically whispered the Painter. Luckily the Professor didn't hear.

The café was not well lighted. At the marble tables stooped the bent backs of old men, men who wore curls over their ears, whose hats were only removed at bedtime. They played chess in the dusk and drank coffee at intervals, regarding their neighbours suspiciously. Rembrandt would have admired the dim, misty corners where on musty divans he could have discerned a head, partly in shadow, a high light on the bridge of the nose, or fingers

snapping with exultation in a sudden shaft of sunlight that came
through a window opening on the west. Groups of two or three
hovered about the players. The stillness was punctuated by street
cries and the occasional rumbling of that ramshackle horse-car
the sight of which sends your wits wool-gathering back to the
'80's.

"Wake up," urged the Painter. "I'm going to sketch that table
in the corner; the two old birds are watching each other as if
plunder were hid somewhere. You know they are afraid to drink
beer because a drop too much might lose them a move. So they
stick to coffee." He went away, the Professor following.

"Is your friend a painter or only one of those newspaper artists
who worry us so much?"

I turned. Besides me sat a mythical old fellow, white-haired,
his coat buttoned to his neck, no shirt, evidently, and the hand
which plucked his beard as white as a girl's—a girl who has white
hands, I mean.

"You look like the Ancient Mariner," I said, "or a Hebraic
Walt Whitman."

He smiled. "I may be both for all you know; but you haven't
answered my question."

He inclined a benevolent ear. I informed him of our mission
and of my disappointment. Again the smile, a smile as ancient as
the world and as fresh as to-morrow.

"It is this way," he confided, and his deep-set eyes sparkled.
"You are an idealist. Wait until you are seasoned by eighty years.
I am eighty, and I've lived on the so-called East Side for sixty of
my years. I speak English better than I do Yiddish, yet to earn
my bread I write Yiddish plays, stories, love-letters, and would
preach if my voice would hold out. I am an ex-rabbi. You know
what a rabbi is; you are old enough. An ex-anything is a mistake
—particularly an ex-dramatic critic or an ex-president."

"You must have seen many changes in your life over here," I
ventured.

"My friend, I have seen many changes, yet nothing changes.
We are born, live more or less unhappily, and die. That's all.
There are more of my co-religionists now than there were when
we first went up the Bowery. Then they pulled my beard and

threw stones at us. Now we live in houses built, perhaps, with those very stones; certainly built by our forbearance. We live—"

He prosed on. He bored me, this octogenarian who resembled both the Ancient Mariner and Walt Whitman. I stopped his rambling by asking: "I suppose the socialists and settlement-workers have greatly improved the East Side?"

He sat up and roared like an approaching earthquake. The chess-players looked at him, shrugged shoulders, and again tackled their problems. The Professor deserted the Painter and tiptoed out to us. The Painter never budged.

"Socialists! What are they? They have stirred up my people with empty words, fine phrases. Oh, the dreamers of the Ghetto. This idea of an earthly paradise you may trace back to the Persians, to the Babylonians, perhaps to the Sumerians. We are always looking for the coming of him who will rescue us. We are the idealistic leaven in whatever national bakery we find ourselves. You Americans are smarter. When the dollars arrive you are satisfied; it is your heaven on earth; but for the poor, who know nothing, have nothing, golden words fill them with hope. Better prisons than those slimy deceptions of socialism. Yes, our girls marry rich goyim, rich gentiles—let a woman alone for finding a tub of butter—and then they come down here, some to live and work—their tongue—and tell more lies to dreamers. Ach! it is awful. And your settlement-workers, the white mice, we call them. They mean well, but they are generally misguided busybodies. They pry, pry, pry, and ask insulting questions. Even if we are poor we are humans; we have feelings too. If a Jew is pious they give him a New Testament. They bore or frighten our wives, though they do a lot of good, helping the hungry poor. Yet children go to school hungry. Don't believe altogether in those sights of big new tenements, playgrounds, public schools; there is a lot of misery on your renovated East Side that your philanthropists never reach, that those funny sociological students never see."

I rose.

"Break away!" said the Painter. "I caught the old prophet in my note-book while he was gassing. Let's get out of here."

I bade farewell to the venerable Jeremiah. He looked sadly

after us. Not a drink, not a smoke—nothing! And all that wisdom dissipated into thin air, or into ears that heeded not. I was glad when we passed through the narrow doorway obstructed by a wretched rubber plant—or was it a hat-rack?

Without the sky seemed rolled back from the roofs and was a deep blue transfused by the citron-tinted afterglow of a setting sun. On the street were the fuliginous oil-lamps of peddlers. The din was terrific; it mingled with the smell of fish, fruit, and grease. A motley mob jostled us from the pavements; the middle was the safest roadway. An old woman who sat combing her thin grey hair directed us westward; we thought we had lost our bearings. Slatternly females chaffered with the Jewish and Italian pushcart men. Their gestures were not unlike; southern Europe and remotest Russia employ the sign language, a voluble digital language it is. Shrieks of laughter and dismay attracted us farther up. A dwarf with a big head and dressed in the uniform of the Salvation Army was hemmed in by half a hundred teasing children of all nationalities. I assure you that I saw white girls with Chinese slitted eyes, little Irish girls with the Hebraic nose curve, Negro boys with straight hair and blue eyes. A vast cauldron— every race bubbles and boils and fuses on the East Side. The children are happy. They are noisy and devilish in their energy. They howled at the dwarf, "Pee Wee!" He was impassive and distributed circulars. In front of a kosher fowl shop another small cyclone was in progress. The place was locked, but in the gaslight we could detect hundreds of chickens hopping over the counter and shelves, and the joy their antics gave the little ones outside was worth a dozen Christmas pantomimes.

"To the Hall of Genius, that's where we are heading, boys!" answered the Painter to a query from the Professor.

I had now become the crusty member of the crowd. I was tired. The coffee at the chess café had given me a headache; besides, things were not exactly going my way. I came out on this expedition prepared to scoff, and while I had not remained to pray, nevertheless was I disappointed. So I irritably inquired: "What Hall of Genius? What new pipe-dream is this?"

Good-temperedly he returned: "It *is* a pipe-dream, and before we go up Second Avenue I want you to see what you can't see anywhere outside Paris."

"The Latin Quarter?" I sneered.

"No; Montmartre. Now just hustle along, please. It is getting late and I'm hungry."

As we entered the hall the buzzing of voices was almost deafening. At least a hundred tables were crowded with men and women. On the balconies were more tables. Everyone was drinking either coffee or beer; the men smoked pipes, cigarettes, with here and there a few cigars. The odour was appalling. I never knew Mother Earth grew such poisonous, weedy tobaccos. We found seats not far from the door.

"It's easier to escape," remarked our guide, philosopher, and friend, "and it's easier to point out the celebrities."

"What celebrities?" faintly inquired the Professor, who was almost a physical wreck.

"Celebrities?" was the response. "Well, I should say. There's enough brains and genius under this roof at the present moment to burn up our universities, our musical conservatories, our paint-pot academies"—here the Painter paused, I fancied maliciously —"our law courts."

"But why, why haven't we heard of these transcendent individuals?" I interposed.

"Over there," continued the Painter, not heeding my question, "over there is a young fellow who has written the best short story since Edgar Poe. It's so good no one dreams of printing it."

"There are a hundred like him who have written the best story since Poe—only they hug the Great White Way," hinted the Professor cynically.

The Painter gave him a sour look.

"Never mind. I'm telling this story. The fellow I mean is bald. That's why he keeps his hat on. But the remnants of his hair are curly."

"I dare him to remove his hat." The Professor it was who spoke. I kicked him under the table.

"That fat youth yonder," tranquilly resumed the Painter, "is a second Ernest Lawson. He never saw a Lawson landscape because he never got farther than Second Avenue. His clothes, as you see, are not suitable; but if he ever starts in painting as he can ("But won't," cruelly intercalated the Professor)—then he may join the Academy."

"Fudge," said I.

"Fudge or not, he is a genius. He works, when he does work, in a carriage factory. His friend is the grandest dramatist of the age, without a Broadway production. It's a pity he can only write in Bulgarian. The woman sitting near him has Duse, Bernhardt, and Nazimova beaten to a pulp as actresses."

The Professor stood up wearily.

"Now I'm going," he said. "I suppose you will show us next the most extraordinary composer on the planet."

"Precisely," acquiesced the Painter. "To your left is a Russian pianist who has the charm of Paderewski, the magic of Joseffy, the technique of Rosenthal, and the caprice of De Pachmann."

We paid the reckoning. Catching our waiter by his tin badge I asked him as my friends moved streetward: "Who are those folks at the next table? Are they poets or painters or musicians?"

"Nichts! Your friend was having fun with you," answered the waiter. "They are nearly all cloakmakers, and work in the neighbourhood."

"Oh, hollow East Side! Oh, humbug Painter!" I ejaculated when we reached Second Avenue and its cool, well-lighted perspectives. The Painter smiled.

"I faked you a bit of the East Side you writing fellows are always looking for. Now for dinner."

We ate paprika-seasoned food to the clangour of the usual gipsy band that never saw the Hungarian Putzta. It was at one of the tinsel Bohemias so plentifully scattered along the avenue. I was better satisfied than earlier in the evening, for I had proved that the old East Side was fabulous. I said as much, and was called ungrateful.

"Isn't it interesting, anyhow?" demanded in unison Professor and Painter.

We were about to part at the corner of the street. It was midnight. Suddenly a thin, scared voice asked us to buy flowers. The girl was small. She wore a huge shawl, and on her head was a shapeless hat over which lolled queer plants. But that shawl! It was fit for her fat grandmother and must have weighed heavily upon her frail shoulders. Her features were not easy to distinguish; her eyes seemed mere empty sockets.

The Painter looked at her.

"What you got under that shawl?" he sharply questioned.

The wretched child shifted her feet. "A pussycat I found on Second Street. I'm taking it home fer me sisters."

We bought her ridiculous flowers and she disappeared.

"A regular Luks," I observed.

"A Luks all right, all right," chimed in the Painter.

We went home.

ACKNOWLEDGMENTS

Harcourt, Brace and World for the selection from Lincoln Steffens

Harper and Row for the selection from Abraham Cahan's *The Rise of David Levinsky*

Helen Hall, Director of the Henry Street Settlement, for the selection from Lillian Wald

Mr. Alfred Rice for the selection from James Gibbons Huneker

Anzia Yezierska for the selection from *Red Ribbon on a White Horse*

Maurice Hindus for the selection from *Green Worlds*

The Macmillan Company for the selection from Morris Raphael Cohen's *A Dreamer's Journey*

Professor W. W. Howells for the selection from William Dean Howells

Greenwich House for the selection from Mary K. Simkhovitch's *Neighborhood*

E. P. Dutton and Company for the selection from Jacob Epstein's *Autobiography*

Cooper Square Publishers, Inc. for the selection from Henry Roth's *Call It Sleep*

Charles Reznikoff for the selection from *By the Waters of Mahattan*

Drawings by Miss G. A. Davis and Joseph Becker, from New York City—The Jewish Quarter on the East Side—scenes in Ludlow Street Market.